THE ULTIMATE IN CALORIE-FREE EATING

Picture a food you have a craving for. Clearly focus on it. Now pick it up, put it in your mouth, and go through all the motions and feelings of eating it. Roll it around on your tongue and experience the taste. Enjoy chewing, sucking, or licking it. Feel it go slowly down your throat. Continue to eat it in your usual fashion until you have had enough or it is gone. Experience feeling full and satisfied.

If done completely and vividly, so that you actually experience eating the food, this trip can be fantastic. It does not mean you will never eat the food in reality—but probably you will eat it less often.

"The mental imagery program used by Dr. Stern is an invaluable tool in a weight control program involving the compulsive eater."

WILMER L. ASHER, M.D.,
Executive Director, American
Society of Bariatric Physicians

MIND TRIPS TO HELP YOU LOSE WEIGHT

FRANCES MERITT STERN, Ph.D., AND
RUTH S. HOCH WITH JEAN CARPER

PLAYBOY
PAPERBACKS

MIND TRIPS TO HELP YOU LOSE WEIGHT

Copyright © 1976 by Frances Meritt Stern, Ruth S. Hoch and Jean Carper

Cover photograph copyright © 1981 by PEI Books, Inc.

Published simultaneously in the United States and Canada by Playboy Paperbacks, New York, New York. Printed in the United States of America. Library of Congress Catalog Card Number: 76-44202. Originally published in hardcover by Playboy Press.

Books are available at quantity discounts for promotional and industrial use. For further information, write to Premium Sales, Playboy Paperbacks, 747 Third Avenue, New York, New York 10017.

ISBN: 0-872-16786-0

First Playboy Paperbacks printing November 1977.
Second printing February 1981.

This book is dedicated to the people
we have worked with, have taught,
and have learned from.

If one advances confidently in the direction of his dreams, and endeavors to live a life which he has imagined, he will meet with a success unexpected in common dreams.

—HENRY DAVID THOREAU

ACKNOWLEDGMENTS

The "trips" in this book, developed by the authors, grew out of our work with clients. A few of the mind trips were suggested to the authors by the experiments and techniques of Joseph E. Shorr, Robert Masters, and Jean Houston, Victor Daniels and Laurence Horowitz, and Frances E. Cheek.

We wish to give special recognition to such diverse theorists as Fritz Perls, Aaron T. Beck, Albert Ellis, Jerome L. Singer, and Joseph Wolpe, whose pioneering work in the varieties of inner experience provided the background for our work on imagery.

A special thanks to Marilyn Mercer and Bruce Milove for their support, and to James Connell and Judy Harris, our tireless research assistants.

We are particularly grateful to our husbands, Floyd Stern and Joseph Hoch, for their unflagging enthusiasm, good humor, and cooperation over and above the call of duty. In addition, we extend our sincere appreciation to the others, too numerous to mention by name, who have influenced and assisted us.

Contents

Part Three. THE MIND TRIPS

PART ONE

It's All in Your Mind

1

ALL POWER TO THE MIND

What is so powerful as the uniquely human ability to imagine—to fantasize, to daydream, to construct in the mind's eye the past and the future? The famous Lascaux cave paintings in France, 14,000 years old, are evidence that mankind has always felt compelled to translate his inner thoughts into concrete symbols. Psychologists know that, in fact, the mind is one vast symphony of underlying fantasies, occurring constantly in such rapid succession that we never notice most of them—only those that surface as the dominant "melody."

We use our waking dreams or fantasies somewhat as we do our night dreams, to resolve emotional conflicts, to give us pleasure, to help shape our destinies through mental visions of the future. Some people fall back on vivid imagery to keep them sane. The former Nazi Albert Speer reports in his book *Spandau* that while in prison after the war, he took mental walking trips throughout Europe, using detailed maps.

We all take trips in our minds—while we are *awake,* as well as while we are asleep, though we may not realize it. Such image-making is not a special talent shared only by a few; it is universal. Dr. Jerome L. Singer, a professor of psychology at Yale University, finds such mental activity "a consequence of the ongoing activity of the brain" and "a fundamental characteristic of man's constitution." If you worry—and who doesn't?—you are engaging in daydreaming by conjuring up a mental picture of what you fear the future may bring. If before an important event you go over your plans in your mind, imagining what you will do, what other people will do, you are "rehearsing" the event in your mind's eye. If you think of the past, you are constructing an imperfect, subjective mental picture of what once happened.

The capacity to visualize is one of the miracles of man's existence, and would not have survived millions of years of evolutionary pressures had it not been of enormous significance. Waking images may, indeed, be fundamental to organizing reality—a means of integrating and making sense of the past, present, and future. Some psychologists believe that no thought occurs in the brain without being preceded by an image, that thinking is actually rapid-fire image-making. In that view, "I think, therefore I am" becomes "I image, therefore I am." It's been noted that some of our greatest scientific discoveries, including ones later expressed in intricate mathematical equations, first appeared to their discoverers in the form of images or symbols.

The way our unconscious communicates with our conscious is not through words, but through symbols and images—what Erich Fromm has called "the forgotten language."

Sometimes the images that float across our consciousness are vague, but with attention it's not difficult to bring them into focus, even guide their development. Only in special states of consciousness—such as can be caused by fatigue, extreme sensory deprivation (being in a dark, soundproof room for several days), drugs, or hypnosis—do waking dreams become spontaneous, seemingly out of control with a will of their own; they intrude upon our perception of reality, and then we call them hallucinations. It's something few people have to worry about.

The mind, with its fantasies, daydreams, mental pictures, or "mind trips," has always ruled man's inner life, and thus his external existence too. The ancient Greeks used mental pictures extensively to construct a system for remembering, much the same way so-called memory wizards do today. And what are the Greek tragedies, and subsequently the Shakespearian plays, and in fact all the novels, plays, paintings, sculpture, architecture, musical compositions, and even political structures ever created but the results of an individual's vivid "mind trip" set to paper?

From what we know, all ideas great and small, from all people great and small, stem from the human ability to form images in the mind. In a broader context, Napoleon said, "Imagination rules the world." Human actions are hampered or constrained only to the extent that individuals fail to exercise their innate ability to image and thus give birth to new and different ways of acting and living.

You have the ability to image. Everyone does, and it is a much more powerful ability than you think.

What we will do in this book is show you how to harness that mental energy to help you deal with one of the problems of living: losing weight. From our experience, we know that what you learn will undoubtedly spill over into other areas of your life— that you will like yourself better and have better control over your life in general. It is not only your body; it is your mind and your way of looking at yourself that will change.

We know that the mind trips we have designed and presented in this book work because they have worked for hundreds of people whom we have helped lose weight through our Institute for Behavioral Awareness. And though we use other techniques too, which will be explained in the book as well, we are increasingly using mind trips because we find them so effective and yet so simple.

Our methods may seem miraculous, but they are not. Everything we do and say is supported by psychological theory and experimentation. What we are doing is very similar to what well-known psychologists have been doing in other areas, with incredible success. Our contribution is that we have adapted the methods to the control of weight.

Both of us have a lifelong interest in weight. Until a few years ago, when we started using our methods, we were both quite overweight, and had been most of our lives. Thus we feel we bring both personal and professional understanding to the problem of overeating. This makes it easier to know what works for us and for our clients—and what will work for you.

A "mind trip" is what in more scientific terms

we call "meta-imagery." "Meta" is the Greek word for "beyond"; "meta-imagery" thus means a higher and more organized form of imagery. Until a few years ago it probably would not have been possible for two people hoping to maintain a credible professional reputation to use imagery for weight loss—whether we called it "meta-imagery" or "mind trips." To much of the psychology establishment, it smacked of the psychedelic culture. Though there was plenty of scientific evidence to justify meta-imagery, it was an idea whose time had not yet come.

Now, many psychologists consider imagery the most exciting field in psychology today. Thanks to new discoveries about the brain and the mind and a burgeoning interest in inner experience, the study of mental images has suddenly become respectable. There's widespread acceptance of the belief that the mind is much more powerful than we ever dared dream. It is the inner experience that counts—that shapes people's attitudes, behaviors, and destinies. The view that for so long held sway, that man is formed only by mechanistic external stimuli over which he has little control, is fast fading. We have entered a new era of humanism—a return to a respect for and study of man's inner self and fantasies as the guiding force in his life.

It is in that spirit that we offer you the mind trips. They are presented with extensive explanations of how to use them in the latter part of the book. However, we feel you will get much more out of them—and be convinced of their potency—if you first read the reasons for the current excitement in the psychological community over the use of mind trips, their scientific basis, and how we arrived at developing and using them in the specialized problem of losing weight.

2

OF RATS AND YOGIS

That mysterious entity known as the mind is so powerful that it can control the body. Proof of that is one of the greatest scientific discoveries of this century.

For years, Western physicians were certain that such physical phenomena as blood pressure, heart beat, and brain-wave activity were automatic, under the control of the autonomic nervous system and immune from the mind's interference. Then in the mid-1960s researchers, notably psychologist Neal Miller, first at Yale and then at Rockefeller University, put an end to that belief through experiments showing that rats could be conditioned to alter their blood pressure, heart beat, kidney functioning, and even blood circulation. Through electrical shocks to the pain and pleasure centers of the rats' brains, Miller and his colleagues induced rats in an hour and a half to alter their heart beats—either slowing the rate down or speeding it up by an amazing 85 beats per minute. More astounding, Miller found the rats could control their blood circulation with some precision; they could direct blood to one ear, causing it to blush, while at the same time pulling blood away from the other ear, causing it to blanch.

These results caused a literal rewriting of the medical textbooks and ushered in a new respect for the power of the human mind.

Of course, Eastern philosophers, hypnotists, and some scientists, through their own experience or experiments, had long recognized such powers of the mind. But it is sometimes jokingly said that in the tradition of American psychology, nothing about man is accepted as true unless it is first proved in animals. Thus, Miller's laboratory confirmations lent respectability to the concept of mind-control functioning and cleared the way for other psychologists to explore the far reaches of the mind. One of the immediate results was the expansion of bio-feedback research, in which a person hooked up to a machine is fed visual and auditory signals whenever he or she alters a physiological function, such as blood pressure, heart beat, or brain waves. The individuals might hear a beep or see the arm on a chart rise or fall whenever they did something—though without knowing what it was—to make the body respond. This is also called "visceral learning."

One of the early experiments came out of the Menninger Foundation in Topeka, Kansas. Dr. Elmer Green and his wife, Alyce, had long been fascinated by the mysteries of the mind and were well versed in the German use of a similar process, called autogenics, and in Eastern philosophy. Quite by chance when they were conducting an experiment one day, they discovered that a woman suffering from migraine headaches could change her blood flow—diverting it from the brain to the outer extremities. When this happened the headache disappeared.

Though no one knows quite why, during a migraine headache the blood vessels dilate in the head and contract in the hands. Thus during a migraine attack, a victim may have cold hands, exhibiting a temperature as low as 70 degrees, which is 20 degrees below normal. If the sufferer can "warm" the hands—that is, get the blood back into them—the whole physiological pattern is disrupted and the headache ceases or is severely diminished.

Consequently, the Greens set up an experiment with migraine sufferers and found to their delight that about two-thirds of their subjects were able to control their own headaches. Some did it through regular bio-feedback equipment which signaled to them when the temperature was rising in their hands. But the Greens did not depend entirely on a mere conditioning mechanism, like the shocks given to Miller's rats, in which the brain somehow creates mysterious changes without conscious thinking. The Greens introduced, so to speak, an element of imagination. They found people could actually abort the migraine headache by saying to the surging blood at the onset of a headache: "Go back down," and imagining it was doing so, like mercury descending in a thermometer. Others, they found, could conjure up vivid scenes in their minds which raised their body temperatures in the right places. For example, they might imagine they were on a warm beach or lying beside a pool with their hands resting in the warm water. And the migraine headache would recede.

What the Greens proved is that the imagination is as powerful in effecting physiological changes in the body as the mysterious auto-functioning responses to the bio-feedback machines. No one knows quite how Miller's rats did it. But we know that humans have the gift of being able to make images in their minds, through which they can at will alter the most basic physiological functioning.

The Greens went on to even more dramatic experiments, proving the potential of the human mind. They hooked Swami Rama, a yogi from India, up to their monitoring equipment. The Swami could effect a 10-degree temperature difference between the thumb side and the little-finger side of his palm. He could also stop his heart from pumping blood for a short time, and produce specific brain wave patterns, as the Greens commanded.

Later, the Greens studied Jack Schwartz, who had come to the United States from Holland in 1957. While the Greens watched, Schwartz stuck a 6-inch-long darning needle completely through the biceps of his left arm, puncturing the skin, muscle, and a vein. When he pulled the needle out, though puncture holes were apparent, there was only slight bleeding for fifteen seconds. The second time he did it, no blood appeared, and he suffered no ill effects, not even infection, even though before the demonstration he had rubbed the needle in bacteria-infested dirt.

When later asked how he did it, as reported in Adam Smith's book *Powers of Mind,* he said it was through imagery. He mentally moved outside himself and looked on his arm objectively as if it were *an* arm, not his, but perhaps that of an inanimate object, such as the arm of a chair. He was totally emotionally detached from the image, and he credited his "subconscious mind" for "allowing" him to do it.

Subsequently, bio-feedback has been used widely with ordinary people to control and study all sorts of physiological processes, including heart beat, skin functioning, blood pressure, and brain waves. It has been found that given proper feedback, a person can mentally locate and cause the electrical firing of a single cell! So great and precise is the body's knowledge of itself.

At least for the moment, such precision, except for a rare few, requires some mechanistic feedback to enable the body to know when it is performing correctly. In many cases, however, psychologists feel the bio-feedback equipment is not needed. People can do just as well by producing images and sometimes body instructions in their minds. For example, Dr. Stern has lowered her body temperature to 96 degrees, as measured by bio-feedback equipment. She does it by taking a mind trip to the North Pole, where she stands shivering in the snow without a coat. She can do it equally well by imaging that she is submerged in ice water or has just stepped out of a bathtub into a cold blast of air. She shows all the signs of being exposed to extreme cold—goose pimples and visible muscular trembling.

All of this demonstrates that there is no duality of mind and body, no physical-psychical split, in which the body operates independently of mind "supervision." The mind and body, at least at this stage of research, seem inseparable, fused in their functioning, with, if anything, the mind as the dominant, controlling force. We may have always suspected this to be true, but it is another thing to have scientific evidence for it.

Even more exciting, if you are practical-minded, is the evidence that a primary way the mind exerts its influence is through explicit fantasies, or constructive daydreams, which so often have been relegated to the world of the impractical. It is almost mind-boggling to realize that those reflections on the mental screen can from all appearances have the same, or nearly the same, impact on the body as do real events. Thus, if an image is experienced vividly enough, the body is fooled; it cannot perfectly detect the difference between a real, or sensory, happening and one that originates inside your brain. *That means that your own mind images, which are under your conscious control, are an enormous source of power within yourself.* And you can *purposefully* use them for many things—including losing weight.

3

HYPNOTISTS AND PRIME MINISTERS

Hypnosis is not new by any means, but it is getting increasing scientific attention, and it offers convincing evidence that the power of the mind extends to projecting images that seem real and superimposing images onto the self which completely change behavior.

In his classic book *Hypnotism,* psychologist G.W. Estabrooks tells how he once gave a tea party in Oxford, England, to which he invited two English friends. During the party the two, under a hypnotic spell, went to the door, ushered in the prime minister of England, and for an hour conducted a witty conversation with him in which they laughed a lot and served him whisky and soda. As it turned out there was no prime minister; the Britishers had been talking brilliantly to an empty chair.

It was a hallucination, in which the figure existed only in the minds of the Englishmen. Yet, out of their memories they had managed to conjure up an image of what a prime minister should be, to the extent of hearing what he said, which in fact was what they were instructing him to say out of their own perceptions of what this fantasy prime minister would say. In other words, the projected prime minister came out of the buried fantasy images of the two hypnotized subjects. The prime minister was their "mental picture."

There have been many substantiated reports—both on stage and in scientific settings—that people under hypnosis can make themselves believe they are other people or animals and act accordingly. For example, by getting down on all fours and barking, if you truly believe inside that you are a dog.

Also classic is the demonstration that a hypnotized person can stiffen his muscles and remain rigid, suspended between two chairs with his head on one, his feet on the other. Someone can sit on his middle without causing him to sag. What this proves is that the muscular system is amazing, and that if you truly believe you can become a bridge, table, or steel beam, your imagination marshals forth all the hithertofore unrecognized physical powers of the body to make it seem so.

More recently, hypnosis has been used to warp a person's sense of time. In one instance, a pianist who had a concert to prepare for practiced two hours under hypnosis and was told by the hypnotist she had practiced eight hours; she felt she had received the full value of eight hours' practice.

As parlor games, some hypnotic demonstrations are not so funny—but it is important to realize that the hypnotist is not the all-powerful person. In fact, a hypnotist cannot make you do anything your imagination cannot conceive of as true. Studies of hypnosis consistently show that the ability to be hypnotized depends on your ability to visualize and internalize for the moment that what the hypnotist tells you is true. If you don't believe that, the hypnosis fails. It only succeeds to the extent that you believe it. Once again, it is your mind and its power that is the determining factor.

You are the person who makes your images, and thus you control your own mind.

4

THE ZEN WAY OF SPORTS

Recently, some tennis instructors, taking their cues from the Eastern philosophy of Zen, have told us we learn tennis all wrong. W. Timothy Gallwey, in his book *The Inner Game of Tennis*, says trying hard is the key to failure, and a nonchalant attitude combined with imagery is the sure way to success. He suggests that before hitting the ball, you visualize where you want the ball to go; your internal computer will then take over and do what is necessary to make the ball go there. The part of the self that performs this feat, he says, does not understand words—only images. For example, if you want a powerful service, don't tell your wrist to snap; get an image in your mind of the wrist snapping, and that will do it.

Does it make sense? Unquestionably. Learning

by such imagery is called "mental practice," and its effectiveness is backed up by psychological research. The only thing that might be said is that the Zen tennis masters aren't taking it far enough. Psychological studies show that to practice tennis you probably don't even need to be on the court. You can practice at home, or wherever you are, by imagining that you are hitting forehands, backhands, and serves, and the chances are the "mental practice" will improve certain aspects of your game perhaps as much as actually playing.

There are many reports in the psychological literature on the value of "mental practice" in sports and games. One study with basketball players showed that those who actually practiced free throws for twenty minutes for twenty days improved their accuracy by 24 percent—and those who practiced the free throws only in their heads improved to nearly the same degree, 23 percent. Many professional golfers say they use imagery as a form of practice by going through a trajectory of the shot in their minds before swinging, both on and off the golf course. Champion chess players and concert pianists have said they improve their performances vastly by practicing games or compositions in their minds.

In an Australian study, young men were taught a specific feat of jumping the high bar. None had done it before, but they were taught the proper movements, and then asked to perform them—that is, "see and feel" them in their minds—for five-minute stretches for six days. When it came time for the actual jump, those who had reported the most vivid imagery were judged the best.

Nobody knows exactly how this works; it could be that when you do something correctly in your mind, your body then models itself after your inner image. What *has* been shown is that during such mental practice the brain is stimulated to cause an electrochemical firing of the same muscles as would be used in actual play—even though you do not feel the muscles move. As we said before, the nervous system is stimulated much the same by an image that originates inside your head as by an event outside your head.

The implications of this are enormous for changing both performance and attitudes and habits. You aren't like a rat in a cage that needs electrical shocks to condition behavior. You can learn habits right in your head. You can forge new neurological pathways through mental practice, by your thoughts and images. You can confront frightening situations in your head without fear of suffering actual consequences. You can rehearse new ways of behaving, and have them "sink in." You can even get "full" by eating in your head, without consuming calories.

Doing something in your head can be just as effective as actually doing it. This, in fact, is part of the reason for the power of the mind trips you will take later.

Since you are the master in your own mind, you can control the images to effect learning effortlessly in your head, and that learning will automatically take over to direct your behavior in real life.

In the early part of the century, a Harvard physiologist, Edmund Jacobson, did some landmark work in the relationship between muscles and the mind. Though much of his work was in relaxation, he was fascinated by the human imagination, and he was the first to provide scientific evidence that the imagination affects the body. He wired his subjects so he could detect when there was electrical activity in their muscles, and then asked them to imagine they were lifting a heavy weight. Though there was no perceptible movement, the imagery set off electrical firing in the very muscle cells that would be required.

Jacobson also had people imagine they were watching a tennis game with the ball bouncing back and forth across the net. He observed that their eyes, though closed during the imaginary scene, moved back and forth under the lids just as if they were watching the real event. After many years of study, Jacobson concluded that he had never encountered a mental activity, as reported verbally by his subjects, that was not accompanied by some neuromuscular activity that could be measured and recorded.

More recently, Laura W. Phillips, at the Institute of Human Behavior in California, reported the same thing. When she asked subjects to imagine they were running their tongues over the cut surface of a lemon, their mouths puckered and some were observed making swallowing motions. When she asked them to recall in vivid detail a time they were embarrassed—or to conceive of an instance where they might be embarrassed—some smiled and others blushed noticeably.

During their imagery, her subjects, who were hooked up to electrodes, registered a response. It was pointed out to them that the imagery caused action in their brains, and a corresponding action in their muscles, even though they were not aware of it. For example, as Phillips noted, if you imagine writing your name with a ballpoint pen, or kicking a ball, and don't move a muscle, nevertheless, if you are totally aware, you can notice a tension in the muscles that would be involved.

The point is that as Jacobson so eloquently
pointed out, the imagination has *energy;* it is not a
vacuum of nothingness in the brain, but actually gen-
erates physical energy in the rest of the body. There
is a physical basis for the imagination. And the potential for using the energy of that imagination is nearly
limitless.

Roberto Assagioli, an Italian psychoanalyst and
the founder of the school of psychosynthesis, in his
book *The Act of the Will* set down the rules or laws
governing the imagination. The first and most basic
law, he says, is: "Images or mental pictures and ideas
tend to produce the physical conditions and the external acts that correspond to them." In other words,
images transform themselves into like actions. "For
example," he says, "images or ideas of courage and
high purpose, used skillfully, tend to evoke courage
and produce courageous acts."

Our private mental images, then, are the source
of all action. And the kind of action produced depends on the kind of images. By deliberately changing the images, you can change your habits, attitudes,
the direction of your life—indeed, that illusionary
thing called fate, which is merely the predictable
outcome of your life based on your ongoing images.

If you can firmly instill new images, new corresponding actions will eventually follow.

You are who you see yourself being.

Think good thoughts and you will become a
good person? Think success and you will become
successful? It is not really that simple. There have
been many popular books on the "power of positive
thinking," and though there is value in thinking positively as opposed to negatively, such advice only
scratches the surface. The problem is not in thinking
positive thoughts, but in *believing* them. A person

does not gain success by imagining he is successful, but by seeing himself doing things that will contribute to his success. The athletes, including the Zen tennis players, do not just use their imaginations to practice; they use their power of imagery.

So far we have used the terms "imagination" and "imagery" as they are commonly used, in some cases interchangeably. But at this point it is important to make a clear distinction between the two.

"To imagine" and "imagination" are rather loose terms, connoting everybody's ability to conjure up images, vague or fleeting, perhaps with little or no conscious attention. They encompass the most undefinable mind wanderings of greater or lesser intensity. Imagining is usually done with the eyes open, and it's often without specific purpose.

On the other hand, "to image" and the corresponding noun "imagery" have a more precise definition as used by psychologists. "To image" means to deliberately call into your mind's eye, with great vividness, an imagined scene or event. It may be something you "remember" or "made up." But to image it is to *experience it at that instant in the present tense* as much as possible—as if you were living it. In imaging you are part of the mental picture. You can see the shapes and the colors, hear the sounds, smell the odors—and, importantly, you can experience your emotions at what you are "seeing." To image successfully you must almost always concentrate deeply and close your eyes to shut out distractions in your environment.

An "image," then, is confined to a specific mental screen through deliberate effort, has more intensity, and demands much more attention than free-floating "imaginary" thoughts.

This is the kind of imagery we mean when we refer to "meta-imagery" and the "mind trips"—a conscious, deliberate act to *create* mind images and guide them.

The images have been lying there for years. And they do not come from anywhere but inside your head. Research shows that the images you see in your mind trips are indeed "memory traces." In other words, at the time you experience an actual event, it is coded in your permanent memory in its entirety—but if asked, you can consciously recall certain outstanding details. However, other parts of the experience of which you were *not* consciously aware are also registered in your memory in amazing detail. And these come out in both guided imagery and night dreams.

The capacity of the human memory is mind-boggling. Everything you ever experienced is recorded on your personal memory tape, and can show up in the mind trips, though you cannot consciously recall it all. The classic evidence of this is the reports of brain probings by a Canadian neurosurgeon, Wilder Penfield, some twenty years ago. During brain surgery under a local anesthesia, when Penfield touched part of the brain with electrodes, his patients burst forth with marvelously detailed accounts of events that had happened years in the past. It was as if they were reliving the event; they spoke of it as happening in the present tense, though they were still aware of being on the operating table. They could hear sounds, smell smells, and experience feelings just as they had at the time of the happening many years ago. The memory tape, in perfect condition, was rerunning. All those hidden feelings and long-forgotten images were still there. Penfield's experiments astounded the scientific community, but his findings are universally accepted. Everything you have ever seen or experienced is still there, still with you, and you can tap that enormous power inside you to explain and change the present.

5

FREUD AND THE EUROPEAN
MIND-TRIPPERS

Until the 1960s, when the California therapists, such as Fritz Perls at Esalen, burst on the scene, psychotherapy in this country paid little attention to fantasies or other waking images in the mind. Therapists were concerned only with night dreams, if with images at all. Their authority, of course, was the Viennese psychoanalyst Sigmund Freud, with his dream analysis and free association.

But in Europe, where Freud's influence was not dominant, therapists were free to explore the meaning of daytime images. Which they did and still do with great enthusiasm. They were influenced by Freud's one-time friend and associate Carl Jung, who was convinced that man lives by his inner images. Jung believed that certain primitive symbols from the "collective unconscious" had a common meaning to all people in a culture, and that waking images were as important as sleeping ones in determining what was going on in the unconscious.

Thus, many European therapists have helped patients become aware of their hidden motivating thoughts by taking them on mind trips, carefully planned and directed by the therapist. The patient is thoroughly awake, but lies down, closes his eyes, and calls forth the images the therapist suggests. As the trip continues the patient reports what is happening to him—what he sees and feels. It is, of course, what one could call an analysis of a waking dream—instead of an analysis of a sleeping dream, which is so common in this country.

These European therapists are convinced that the same unresolved conflicts appear in your waking dreams as in your night dreams. But during the waking dreams, *at the time they are happening,* a skilled therapist can guide you in understanding and resolving them, by making suggestions from the sidelines for new directions in the waking dreams.

For example, if you are walking through a meadow and you meet a frightening image, such as horse, giant, or monster that is symbolic of unresolved fears, it might be wise to "face it down"— that is, stand up to the frightening image and overcome it. Or it may be better at that time, as Hanscarl Leuner, the German pioneer in waking-dream therapy, suggests, to disarm it subtly by trying to make friends with it or feeding it. Leuner suggests that you offer food to your fantasy monster, and feed it until it becomes overstuffed and falls asleep. An odd fate for a "vicious" monster.

Even Freud at one time used the analysis of waking fantasies in his practice. He told of bringing out "pictures and ideas" by means of pressing on the patient's head. He took the patient's head between his hands, and told the patient he would "see something in front of you or something will come into your head" and "it will be what we are looking for." Freud was amazed to note that while awake, but with eyes closed, a woman patient reeled off scenes pertinent to a central problem, in succession, as if she were "reading a lengthy book of pictures whose pages were being turned before her eyes." Still, Freud went on to lose interest in such therapeutic imagery, and it was not exported to America until the 1960s, though it has been used routinely in Europe for fifty years or so.

Today, nothing is generating so much interest among psychologists, psychiatrists, and the self-appointed gurus of the human-potential movement as the constructive use of imagery. "Guided imagery" is still hardly a household word or a staple in every therapist's closet of "cures." But even some conventional therapists are finding it easier to get at the patient's unconscious through a complete guided daydream, enacted in front of him, than through half-forgotten dream fragments. What some consider to be the *most* successful therapy ever developed— that of desensitizing patients to their phobias and irrational fears—has as its very core extensive visualization of the phobia itself. And there is not a single new therapy among the many proliferating ones that the authors can think of that does not use guided imagery of some sort.

Youngsters are getting boosts in their self-esteem through guided imagery. People are losing fears, getting in touch with themselves, bringing deeply buried problems into their awareness, and

ridding themselves of all kinds of undesirable habits
—in fact, transforming their lives—through this new
method, which now is found in this country under
half a dozen different names: guided fantasy, inner
imagery, active imagination, the directed daydream,
mental imagery, guided affective imagery, waking-
dream therapy. Ten years ago one could hardly find
two or three references to imagery in that monthly
Bible of current information, *Psychological Ab-
stracts*. Today, each edition carries fifty or so. It's as
if, after thousands of years, imagery has been rescued
from the realm of poets and mystics and put into the
realm of science. What for laymen has been common
sense all along, that man's destiny is shaped by his
dreams, is now recognized and supported scientifically.

Much of the current interest in guided daydream therapy comes from the Italian Assagioli, the
German Leuner, and a Frenchman, Robert Desoille.
Of these, Assagioli has probably had the most influence in this country, because his work is widely available in translation. But it is Desoille who was the
frontrunner in developing the therapeutic use of
"waking daydreams" in a highly structured way. He
took several basic themes he felt were common to all
people (reminiscent of Jung's symbols of the collective consciousness) and had the patient build image
trips around them. For example, he had the person
descend to the depths of the ocean; ascend a mountain; descend into a cave; seek out a wizard, witch, or
magician; search in the forest for the castle of "Sleeping Beauty." Desoille and his followers felt that skillfully conducted inner explorations of these universal
themes would help a person work through his basic
conflicts. The European therapists have reported

amazing successes. Leuner, for example, reported that with "guided affective imagery" he could drastically reduce the time needed for the treatment of neurosis (he made no claims for psychosis) from an average of 160 hours for conventional "talk therapy" to an average of 40 hours of "imagery therapy."

It's apparent that through structured mind trips the patient short-circuits the usual communication systems, by going directly to the unconscious or other levels of awareness. Therapists, both here and abroad, are constantly amazed at what a shortcut imagery is, at how quickly it can reveal hidden meanings and identify problems—which become *instantly* clear to the dreamer. For example, Martha Crampton, at Sir George Williams University in Montreal, tells of a woman who was asked to visualize her relationship with her husband. In a flash, the woman saw herself as a tiny frightened helpless bird, held tightly in a clenched hand. At the therapist's suggestion, the woman made the hand open so the bird could fly away. Eventually "the bird" made it to an island where she found seeds—that is, sustenance —on her own. This one mind experience, Crampton says, radically improved the woman's relationship with her husband.

Unlike traditional therapy, guided imagery usually requires no discussion between therapist and patient to make the point clear. As Desoille noted, the trips themselves are intrinsically curative.

Further, the guided trips allow the individual to exercise immediate and firm control over the situation. Through a dramatic confrontation with the images, a person may symbolically overcome them, come to terms with them, or defuse them of meaning. How threatening can a symbolic monster be, if you can overcome it by stuffing it with cookies?

Sometimes there is an infusion of myth and magic that gives the dreamer symbolic control. Suppose in your fantasy you meet a monster in a grotto? One way to deal with it is to touch it with a magic wand—which causes it to reveal its *true* identity. Desoille says the monster then is likely to turn into the person the monster symbolizes for you in real life.

Once aware, you can go on to deal with it in real life; recognition of the emotional obstacle is the first step to change, in any therapy.

It's fascinating to note that people deal with their fantasies, or guided daydreams, much the same way they deal with real life. When asked to climb a mountain in his mind, a person who can't seem to succeed in real life may find his way strewn with rocks and other obstructions he can't get around. However, therapists find that in guided daydreams, patients can overcome the obstacles, through many imaginative techniques, such as having a bulldozer come and thrust a rock aside or having a helicopter come over and carry it away, clearing the path. The theory, as proved by experience, is that if you can do it symbolically, you markedly increase your prospects of actually doing it.

If you can get rid of the "rocks" in your images, you clear the way for success in real life.

All the time you are on the mind trip, you are learning, and that learning will be transferred to real life. You discover that you are in control of the images; you can make them do as you want—and similarly you can make your real life go where you want. You are not really beleaguered by circumstances beyond your control; you are in control.

6

A BIT OF THE HAIR
OF THE DOG . . .

Since therapy is usually an art, much of its effectiveness goes unproved, and to some it may seem fanciful. But nothing could be more hard-headed, scientifically proved, or remarkable than the results American therapists have had in ridding people of their fears by applying imagery—and what *Psychology Today* magazine has called "a bit of the hair of the hound." Through structured mind trips, therapists have achieved undreamed-of but undisputed success in ridding people of all types of phobias and irrational fears.

The technique is called systematic desensitization. The theory is that if you give a person a little bit of his phobia in small, controlled doses, it will lose its power to affect him. It is the same principle as gradually accustoming a frightened child to water by letting him approach the water, stick in his toe, and then wade in.

Since it is impractical to bring patients in contact with their real fears—snakes, spiders, heights, elevators, etc.—or to control the anxiety produced by actual encounters, patients are asked to confront their phobias by imaging them. They image long scenes in which they gradually see, approach, then confront the feared object, until it becomes nonthreatening.

Obviously, the true test of the method is whether the desensitization in the mind carries over to real life. If you learn to look a snake in the eye in your head, can you do it in the real world? No question. The number of people who have walked out of their therapists' offices and confronted their phobias without trembling are legion. Many had seemed totally hopeless cases.

The father of this therapy, Joseph Wolpe, in one study reported that through systematic desensitization, 90 percent of the fears were completely eliminated or markedly decreased (to the extent the patients judged them to have lost 80 percent of their potency). The phobias Wolpe successfully treated included fears of confinement, storms, examinations, snakes, being watched, disapproval, crowds, criticism, bright lights, palpitations, blood, elevators. Others have confirmed Wolpe's findings and added to the list to include almost any anxiety-producing situation you can imagine—being alone at night, being in the dark, writing reports, making speeches, failing sexually. Anything considered to have an element of the phobic can be treated by such therapy.

At the heart of the therapy is the patient's willingness and ability to image. For, as Wolpe notes, a person who fears dogs gets just as anxious imagining he's meeting one as he does actually confronting one. During the sessions the patients often cry, scream, or tremble, exhibiting all the physical and emotional reactions of an actual encounter.

First, the therapist has the person close his eyes, and relax as completely as possible. Relaxation is considered by Wolpe to be crucial to the results. You can't be relaxed and anxious at the same time. Others believe, also, that it is much easier to produce vivid imagery when relaxed because you block out distractions. The therapist then presents scenes involving the phobia, which the patient images. The imagery is usually meticulously scaled, starting with scenes that produce the least anxiety and building to those that produce the most. Thus, through imagery, the patient and therapist can control the amount of anxiety generated. If a scene becomes too threatening for the person to handle at the moment, he can easily end it. Also, imagery entails no potentially dangerous consequences, such as actually being bitten by a dog.

If a patient were being desensitized to snakes, here is a typical high-anxiety scene he might be asked to image, as described by Milton Wolpin, at the University of Southern California, who has used the method extensively.

"Close your eyes. Imagine yourself getting up out of the chair in which you are now sitting. Picture yourself walking across the room, opening the door, and walking out into the corridor. Visualize yourself walking along the corridor to the stairs. Imagine yourself now leaving the building and starting to walk across the grounds to the building where the snake is housed. Picture yourself opening the door to the room where the snake is. Imagine going in, closing the door, and looking across the room, where you see the snake in its cage. Picture yourself now walking across the room. Imagine that you get closer and closer to the cage until you are standing next to it. Visualize yourself putting your hand on the cover at the top of the cage. Imagine removing it. Now picture yourself standing there and reaching into the cage. Image that your hands are just above the snake and that you see the snake moving. Imagine now that your hands close gently but firmly around the snake. Picture yourself picking it up and removing it from the cage. Imagine that you have the snake in your hands and that you are holding it next to your body. Picture yourself walking over to a chair and sitting down on it. Imagine that as you sit there you put the snake in your lap and you allow it to crawl around; imagine that you have removed your hands from the snake and that you are watching it crawl around in your lap. Notice how it moves around, crawling here and there. See how it sticks its tongue out and how it moves its head about. Suppose now that the snake has been in your lap for a while and crawling about some. Imagine now that once again you put your hands firmly but gently around the snake. As you hold it in your hands you stand up and walk over to the cage. Imagine now that you are putting the snake back in the cage. Now picture yourself putting the cover onto the cage. Imagine now that you leave the snake in the cage, leave the room, and walk back across the grounds to the building from which you had just come. Okay. Open your eyes."

If you read that scene carefully, and go through it in your mind, you will understand its power. It seems that you are actually going through the motions of handling and experiencing the snake. Even reading it slowly with eyes open has some impact.

But the greatest effect comes when the person gets intensely into the scene. Jerome Singer in his book *Imagery and Daydream Methods in Psychotherapy and Behavior Modification* notes: "The therapist has to be sure the patient is not simply saying the words that are associated with the frightening event. If the patient merely thinks verbally 'little dog barking' and does not generate a fairly complete picture of the dog barking and perhaps even have an auditory image of the sounds of the barking along with the picture of the dog, it is possible the effect will be essentially 'lip service.' "

In the most vivid effective imagery, you not only *see* what is going on, you experience it with all your senses.

How does it work? Why does it work? Since the mind's functioning, despite ongoing research, is still mysterious, no one knows for sure. There are various explanations: that the imagery is counterconditioning, much as you could use on a rat in a laboratory; that it is "rehearsal" or "mental practice," much as the golfers use; that it involves learning through "modeling," in that you see yourself performing, and then imitate your actions in real life.

Some also believe that just controlling the images in the mind gives many patients a thrill—a real boost of self-esteem and accomplishment—and they realize for the first time that they can control their lives and fears. This produces a good feeling that then further reinforces their desire and abilities to be in control.

It is probably a combination of all of these, with perhaps some unknowns thrown in. *How* it works is uncertain. That it *does* work is certain.

7

MIND TRIPS
MADE POPULAR

If you look in on almost any new type of therapy or on consciousness-raising sessions of the "human potential movement," you might see people deep in mind trips, talking to chairs, or otherwise acting out their fantasies. For example, Werner Erhard's est (Erhard Seminars Training), a nationwide organization which claims to train people in "aliveness," makes extensive use of "processes," which are prolonged imaging directed by a group leader. "Psychodrama" is the acting out of fantasies and coming to grips with them. The Gestalt therapists depend on imagery, as does Transactional Analysis to a lesser extent. Taking mind trips can also be pure fun, as Robert Masters and Jean Houston explain in detail in their book *Mind Games*.

Thus, the kind of mind trips, therapeutic or

otherwise, are a far cry from Desoille's classic few.

If you have a headache you might be asked to visualize it. What color is it? How big is it? Where is it in your head?

You have a conflict to work out? See each hand as a warring faction of yourself. Then have the hands talk to each other. What do they say?

You have a worry you don't like? Image it in your hand, and then symbolically give it away.

Image you are an inanimate object—a fruit, a vegetable, a tree, a rock. What does it feel like? What do you say?

Explore your body. Go in your mouth, proceed down through the digestive tract, noticing everything. What do you find?

Go inside your head. What do you find there?

On a more existential level, if you are troubled about your deepest concerns in life, image going into a cave or to the top of a mountain where you meet a wise man. Ask him a question about life, and see what he answers.

Mind trips like these are being used widely now to help people expand their awareness as well as to combat specific problems.

One of the most imaginative users of mind imagery for a specific purpose is Joseph E. Shorr at the Institute for Psycho-Imagination Therapy in Los Angeles. Shorr uses imagery not only to get people to recognize inner conflicts but also to change their self-concepts by "working through" what he calls "task imagery." Shorr has people image that they build a bridge across a gorge, build a house, walk away from a plane crash, climb 1,000 steps, or perform other demanding tasks. How a person approaches such a task in his mind reveals much about his life style, problem-solving patterns, and personality.

Some might start with energy and soon give up. One person might build a swinging rope bridge; another, one of steel girders. Some builders encounter difficulty in construction immediately; others have their project collapse just as they are about to complete it. Or a typhoon might come along and wipe out all the work. Whatever the imagery, Shorr says it is rich, remarkable, and reveals a life view. More important, he finds that a meaningful mind struggle in which the self-defeating forces are vanquished and the task is successfully completed can be a catalyst for real life success.

In his book *"Psychotherapy Through Imagery"* he tells of a man who, when asked to climb 1,000 steps, remained stuck on the 995th step, hanging on in fear and trembling. Only at Shorr's urging could the man get up courage to try to go farther; finally, after much struggle, he made it to the top, and it represented a great victory. The man had always thought of himself as "second best"—a person who did not want to alienate others while getting ahead. After conquering the step-climbing in his mind, Shorr says the man went on in his profession to assume a "first position." But Shorr doesn't think he could have done it had the internal struggle during the imagined climb not been so intense, so real.

8

YOU CAN TURN YOURSELF ON —OR OFF—ANYTHING

A half-century ago, the psychologist J.B. Watson conditioned a three-year-old boy to be afraid of rabbits. A little later another psychologist deconditioned a little boy of his fear of rabbits. Both did it through manipulating stimuli and responses. Ever since, psychologists have been experimenting with changing behavior through deliberate reward and punishment: reward, of course, to promote desired behavior, and punishment to deter it. The press has reported many such efforts, notably electric shocks and other painful administrations to "modify" behavior. Fortunately, much of that kind of experiment is out of fashion today, considered objectionable and in some instances inhumane.

Still, the principle of altering behavior by reward/punishment is valid, and can be used more gently and effectively. Your own images can, and do, act as rewards and punishments and are instantly on call. It's something many successful and unsuccessful people automatically do to monitor their actions, though they aren't always aware of it.

As we grow up we learn, often haphazardly through accidental associations. If you have ever been sick after eating a certain food, or having too much to drink, or experiencing any other profoundly unpleasant or sickening event, you know how long it is before you can face that food or similar situation again without a feeling of nausea or revulsion. Often just the thought of it can turn you off.

If this can happen accidentally, it can also be made to happen intentionally. All you have to do is bring to mind a sickening image and associate it with an unwanted habit. You don't have to actually experience the habit or the sickness. All you have to do is create the scene in which you participate in the undesirable activity, and then immediately get sick, all in your mind.

In the mid-1960s the psychologist Joseph Cautela began using such "aversive" image therapy to help people get rid of unwanted traits and habits, such as compulsive stealing, homosexuality, obesity, and alcoholism. Cautela first had the patient "approach" his vice in his mind, by imaging opening the refrigerator door, or stepping up to a bar, or accosting a person of the same sex. The scene then turns ugly and repulsive. For example, in the case of alcoholics, Cautela had them image that after they had had a few drinks at a bar, they vomited all over it and themselves. After the scene is played out and the person is sufficiently repulsed, he immediately shifts to a pleasant scene in which he feels good, as a reward.

Cautela and others have been quite successful, especially with alcoholics. One study showed 100 percent success, with all of the subjects on the wagon after eight to fifteen months. Aversive images have also worked well for smoking and obesity.

Though nausea and vomiting are the images of choice, anything sufficiently repellent or frightening will work. Television news director Earl Ubell in his book *How to Save Your Life* says he automatically dropped weight through aversive thoughts. Every time he was faced with fattening foods, the dead face of his overweight father, who had died of a heart attack, flashed into his mind.

The psychological literature is full of cases proving the success of noxious imagery. It is powerful. However, equally powerful is positive imagery. In fact, there is sufficient reason to believe that positive images are more potent in shaping behavior than negative ones, just as it has been established that rewards are more influential than punishment. That is why it is important with noxious mind trips to end the scene by switching to a positive image, as Cautela does. It is not reinforcing to end the scene with a bad feeling that comes from imagined nausea. If you make yourself sick with such images, you should also give yourself a bromide to feel better. Also, we find some people are reluctant to participate in noxious imagery if they are left with no relief and an unpleasant feeling. It's essential to always follow up a negative mind trip with a positive one.

Positive images can heighten your spirits, act as powerful internal reinforcers, and spur you on to greater achievements. Cautela, for example, ha taught people to carry around a positive image which they can pull out in case of "emergency" to deter undesired actions. When faced with a persistent problem, the person first flashes a positive predetermined thought in his mind, such as "I can do that," and follows it up instantly with an image that shows him or someone else doing it. Cautela found in some cases it's even more effective to call forth an image of another person performing as you would like to perform. That's called "modeling," patterning your behavior after someone you admire.

Commonly Cautela has people flash into their minds a movie screen on which a film is in progress. One of Cautela's cases was a woman who used to get in violent arguments with her husband. When that was about to happen, she imaged a movie screen with a woman sitting calmly, undisturbed, while her husband raved at her. Thus she learned to remain calm too in such circumstances.

The joy of positive mind trips is that they can be produced whenever you need them. One woman in our program imagines after doing something she is proud of that a big velvet glove comes out of the sky and pats her on the back. Mrs. Hoch rewards herself with pleasant mind trips that take her to her "favorite place," which is a resort in the mountains. You can use such positive mind trips for any number of things: to relax in the dentist's chair, to endure hectic traffic (when someone else is driving), to take your mind off food. Many people in our program, when they feel the urge to eat, instead take a mind trip; often they flash into their minds a thinner image of themselves which they foresee for the future. The image acts both as an incentive, moving them toward their vision, and as an instant mental reward for not eating.

At first, while you're learning, such images must be repeated. After practice, you can flash them into your mind any time you need them—wherever you are.

Feeling good has more power than feeling bad.

9

YOU ARE WHO YOU SAY YOU ARE

From the time you are born you probably engage in an internal dialogue in whatever language is appropriate. You pick up signals from your environment and the people around you about what kind of person you are. You absorb or internalize the statements about yourself, then you feed them back to yourself —forever! Unless you change the tape in your head, so to speak. What you think about yourself determines your self-image and your self-instructions, or how you tell yourself to behave. And you cannot for long act contrary to your own self-image. That self-image carries with it what Prescott Lecky, a pioneer in self-image psychology, called the concept of "the consistency of the personality." In short, if you believe you cannot learn, it will be inconsistent with your self-image to do so. Similarly, if you believe you cannot lose weight, and have failed numerous times in the past, it will be inconsistent for you to do so on any lasting basis, unless you become aware of those deeply hidden self-defeating self-statements you are making, and correct them.

Otherwise, you continue to act on the self-statements, though you have long ago forgotten what they are. Carl E. Thoresen of Stanford University, the co-author of a wonderful book called *Self-Control: Power to the Person,* points out that people very early become deaf to their own self-statements. He explains: "The young child talks aloud to himself at first and then gradually replaces these overt verbalizations with covert talk or self-verbalization, in the form of self-instructions. After the first few years of life, the person engages in a great deal of covert (internal) speech . . . However, his awareness of this internal behavior quickly diminishes. Thus, over time it *seems* to the person as if what he does is spontaneous and totally determined from within." At that point, you no longer hear the internal voices, but you still obey them.

Further, it is a vicious circle. How you behave, based on your learned self-image, sets up expectations in others, either positive or negative. How they then expect you to behave is how you *do* behave. It becomes a self-fulfilling prophecy. Studies have shown that children perceived of as intelligent, and told so, get better grades. The psychologist Kenneth Clark points out the self-fulfilling effects of prejudice. If you are viewed and treated as inferior you are likely to act in ways to conform to that precept.

We often see people who lose weight and are no longer "fat," though they still see themselves as fat and refer to themselves as fat. (And interestingly, slim people can gain weight to the point they are no longer considered slim—yet they still think of themselves as thin, and tend to underestimate their true body size.) To illustrate: One woman who lost 30 pounds in our program went shopping for a new pants suit, but everything she tried on did not look as good as she had imagined—the pants were baggy and the jacket hung loosely. Not until Mrs. Hoch pointed out a person in a shopping center who resembled the woman in size could she get her image of her body shape in tune with reality. She had been trying on size 14; when she mentally realized she was smaller, she shopped for a size 12 and found one that fit perfectly.

It's true, as we and other researchers have found, that many overweight people feed themselves negative self-statements. They say internally or aloud: "I'm a pig." "I'm a big fat cow." "I'm stupid because I can't lose weight and keep it off." "I'm weak." "I have no will power." "I'm a failure." "I'm a worthless person." "Everyone is more beautiful, talented, and happy than I am." In fact, a prevalent myth among the overweight is that all thin people are happy per se. This is dangerous, for it sets you up for failure if you get thin and happiness doesn't appear at your doorstep. It means you have linked all your problems to your weight, and though that may be a contributing factor to unhappiness, it is rarely the whole cause. Getting thin, per se, will not give you a new self-image. It is the other way around:

Give yourself a new self-image and you will get thinner.

One of the most exciting recent discoveries is that destructive self-statements that contribute to faulty self-images can be changed through repetition and imagery. Remember that statement of Coué's: "Every day in every way I am getting better and better"? Though it often produces snickers among so-called sophisticates, current psychological research shows it is not off base. Repetition of more positive self-statements, followed by reinforcing images, can change behavior. However, two things are necessary: First, you must eventually internalize them so they become automatic, absorbed by your unconscious; and second, in order to do that, you must believe they have a basis in credibility. If a person of average looks repeats over and over, "I am as beautiful as Miss America," it is not likely to "take" and become integrated because the contrary feedback from others would be too great.

The purpose of modifying your self-statements is to give you self-control.

Hypnotists often use what they call the "ten-finger exercise." Just before going to sleep, you repeat in your mind ten times, counting off a finger each time, some positive statement to change yourself. For example, "I am becoming more and more attractive." "I am losing interest in smoking." "I am eating less and liking myself more."

The reason for doing it before sleep is that your resistance if you are relaxed is much less, and the repetition may act as a kind of posthypnotic suggestion. However, combining suggestion with *images* of yourself acting the way you describe yourself adds untold potency to the effectiveness. In fact, the fingers and counting may only act as a framework for implanting the images. Some therapists say if you go to bed with an image of yourself jumping out of bed in the morning with zest, the chances of its happening are increased. Dr. Stern, when she has extensive work to complete, repeats at bedtime, "My energy level is rising" ten times, and images herself in a Wonder Woman suit, going about the tasks in a whirlwind. When she did it over a three-week period, her productivity markedly increased.

In another remarkable instance, illustrating the power of self-statements and what happens when you change them, one woman in our group used mind trips to change her self-image; she lost 45 pounds, and now has a confident, self-assured, very attractive self-concept, and is one of our group leaders. However, her eight-year-old daughter, Jill, was doing miserably in school. The little girl was leaving notes for her parents that read: "Jill is dumb. Jill is ugly. Jill has no friends," etc.

Our group leader had the little girl practice new positive self-statements every night. She also had her go through imaging that she got up, went to school, met her friends, sat down at her desk, listened to the teacher, and took a spelling test, or whatever was happening the next day. She "rehearsed" the event in her mind; she mentally practiced doing well on the tests.

After three weeks, her grades improved remarkably, and the teacher said it was a "miracle." Jill also started leaving notes that revealed a transformed opinion of herself. They now read: "Jill is a smart little girl." She has now also started saying aloud the same things about herself and *believing* them.

Psychologist Albert Ellis has pioneered in getting people to listen to the irrational self-statements that control their lives, and to give them up and replace them with more realistic self-statements. Donald Meichenbaum, at the University of Waterloo in Ontario, Canada, also has conducted investigations into what people say to themselves and has found ways to change them. He taught hyperactive and impulsive children to "think aloud" and give themselves instructions which calmed them down. He taught schizophrenics to give themselves instructions, such as "I will be relevant and coherent and make myself understood." In other instances, mental patients have greatly improved by being told "to act like normal people." Apparently by copying normal behavior or "modeling," they internalized their new ways, perhaps the same way athletes unconsciously improve by watching and mentally imitating better players.

Much of Meichenbaum's success is due to mind-trip "rehearsals" of proper behavior. One of his findings is fascinating: If you image self-instructions *before* the actual event, you're more likely to carry them out than if you actually give yourself the instructions at the time of the act. In short, *image* that you are on a basketball court where you tell yourself to "make that basket." Or *image* that you open the refrigerator door and tell yourself to close it and not eat anything. That is more effective in guaranteeing that you carry out the self-instructions than if at the time you actually open the refrigerator door you say to yourself: "Shut the door and don't eat anything." Such mind practice has an amazing ability to strengthen your psyche's ability to take you in the direction you want to go.

Studies repeatedly prove that if you are afraid of doing something, or say you "can't" do something, such as make speeches, take tests, be creative, or lose weight, it is likely that you are making silent deprecating self-statements and giving yourself instructions that destine you for failure in that area. If you can ferret out the negative statements and replace them with positive, success-oriented ones, you will no longer be afraid or "unable" to make speeches, take tests, be creative, or lose weight. You will be more apt to succeed at whatever you do.

Your mind is a rich, awesome storehouse of images, answers, and solutions. If you are overweight it is your mind that is defeating you. For the body goes as the mind directs. To lose weight permanently, then, you must literally change your mind. You must enter fully into yourself, into your inner resources. For even though you may not realize it, you have all the answers inside you; it is a question of releasing them and restructuring them. You do know what is best for you, but somewhere along the line, you internalized certain attitudes toward food, a style of eating, and consequently some self-concepts and images about food that continue to direct you. When you change those, and only when you change those, will you find a permanent solution to your weight.

Now, just as we gave you scientific evidence for the power of mind trips, we want to tell you a little about current research about overeating and our philosophy of losing weight. You will then be in a perfect position to see how the mind trips are styled to mesh with all these concepts. It is important that you do, for the more strongly you believe the mind trips will work for you, the more effective they will be.

PART TWO

Why You Can't Stop Eating

10

THE MYTH OF WILL POWER

Being overweight, by a little or a lot, is not a moral problem. It is not a reflection on your character; nor is it a sign of a weak will. It has nothing to do with your constitution, nor your endocrine system (except in rare cases). Most important, the psychological literature on overweight and obesity shows that heavier people are no more neurotic than other people.

Most people who overeat have no idea why they do so. Many no sooner have eaten the last bite, than they say to themselves: "Now why did I do that?" It is almost as if someone has given you a posthypnotic suggestion, which caught you unawares but nevertheless was something you felt compelled to obey. To an extent that is very close to the truth. You have a lifetime accumulation of responses to food that run in your head like a tape, over and over. Numerous studies show that overweight people often respond differently to food than normal-weighted people; such responses cause you to follow inner urgings probably developed in childhood that are now grooved into the mind. They are now consolidated into patterns of eating. And they are obstacles to permanently losing weight.

Unfortunately, the American way of dieting rarely takes these powerful forces into consideration. And that is why weight loss is generally such a failure.

One of the most depressing things about opening any book on obesity is that it invariably starts off with the news that the malady is virtually "untreatable." That means many physicians, psychiatrists, and lay groups have had only moderate success. Further attesting to the extent of failure is the number of crash diets that come on the market every year. It is painful to watch Americans switch hopefully from one diet to another, each one with some medical underpinnings guaranteeing success. For it is invariably futile; the pounds disappear but quickly reappear when the diet has ended. Almost all such weight-loss programs depend on two factors with built-in failure: diet and its taskmaster, will power. But those who concentrate on treating overweight as if it were a moral problem, which only a stiffening of will power is needed to overcome, are neglecting the conflicting power of the person's inner life.

Will power will not work.

Will power, in fact, is self-defeating, for in the conventional meaning, it demands 100 percent compliance. And though a few rare people are able to accomplish that, most are not. Even a minor infraction, then, fills you with feelings of inadequacy, even anger and self-disgust. These negative feelings in turn set you up for further defeat, and eventually, faced with constant failure and guilt, you stop trying.

It was the Frenchman Emile Coué who said that when the imagination is in conflict with the will, as we conceive of it, the imagination will win out every time. It is true. For nothing is so powerful as those images etched in your mind, and no matter how hard you try, you cannot suppress them for long. You may temporarily subdue your inner urgings with so-called will power, but eventually they will reemerge. You cannot permanently shackle, beat, or otherwise intimidate yourself into submission. In fact, such a view of will power is a misconception.

Assagioli, who spent many years contemplating the nature of the will, has said that the Victorian concept of the will as something stern, repressive, and forbidding is in truth a caricature of the will. He says there is no will so potent that it can *force* you to accomplish something if it is against your "true personality drives." The true purpose of a will, in Assagioli's view, is not to exert such power, but to gently organize and carry out directives of the inner self. In short, your will must be in line with the desires and motivations of your inner world, or you will not succeed over the long run.

Studies on permanent weight loss have shown that "will power" is hopelessly ineffective compared with actually changing patterns of eating. Other evidence shows that deliberately refraining from a bad habit can backfire and reinforce it, making it stronger and harder to break. Interestingly, the Greens and other experimenters with bio-feedback consistently reported that the harder subjects tried to regulate blood pressure, etc., the less successful they were. Exerting so-called will power had the opposite of the desired effect. Only when subjects relaxed and let the control "happen" did they succeed.

When you truly get in touch with yourself, your inner feelings and bodily needs, overeating will not be a problem. Many people who have participated in mind trips report their appetite automatically turns off—that they often lose interest in food, and their body seems to stabilize at a comfortable weight. There is such a thing as inner body wisdom, and you can achieve it.

Overeating is learned and can be unlearned.

Interestingly, there is no evidence that people who remain thin use will power to control their overeating; it is something that seems to come from inside the body—they seem to have mind mechanisms that tell them to shut off food. And they do it, without thinking or agonizing over it. This is not the result of some constitutional superiority. It is the way they have learned to treat food. And the patterns are so deeply ingrained that the behavior takes care of itself, without constant conscious regulation.

Gaining this same kind of control over your body and eating is not at all out of reach. In fact, it is imperative, if you want long-lasting success at losing weight. And you can do it through the power of the mind and the mind trips we have designed specifically for that purpose. If mind trips can cure people of such incapacitating problems as phobias, serious neurosis, smoking, nail biting, impotence, overdependence, and all other such ills of mankind, they can surely have a powerful effect on your ability to lose weight.

If you are overeating, it is not that you cannot

learn; you have already learned very well. It is simply that you have learned the wrong way. You are a great success at what you are doing—namely, overeating. You can also be a success at undereating, and then at eating just enough to keep yourself at a desired weight.

In our program, we do not dwell on negative feelings or do anything to promote defeat. The whole emphasis is on helping a person develop positive feelings toward the self, and thus a positive attitude toward future success. We find that will power and *restrictive* diets are self-punishing and promote negative feelings of deprivation, frustration, defeat, and powerlessness. People on such regimens do not learn new eating patterns to replace old ones for that day the diet ends, as it always must.

11

DIETS: DOOMED TO FAIL

Losing weight is not a problem for most people. Almost everyone who comes into our program has lost hundreds, sometimes thousands, of pounds during a lifetime. The problem, of course, is in not regaining it. Restrictive dieting is an artificial situation which cannot endure in most people's regimens; it is disruptive of the regular routines of living and eating. By drastically altering eating patterns for a short time, people can lose weight, but once the diet ends, the former eating habits resume and predictably produce the same results as before: overweight.

The key to permanent weight loss, then, is to learn new patterns of eating to keep overweight from recurring. People know this instinctively, but do not know how to do it; they do not know how to change those mysterious drives that keep them fat, nor unlock the powers that seem to keep others thin. As news of our program has spread, we receive letters from people throughout the country, attesting to this truth. Here are some of them:

"I have lost over 100 pounds. But am having a very hard time keeping from gaining. I don't want to be fat and I know eating will make me fat again, but I eat anyway—and anything."

"I am a member of Tops Club (Take Pounds Off Sensibly), an international organization, and have been for 10½ years. In this time I have at one time lost 81 pounds to my goal and on numerous times after regaining, lost 50 to 60 pounds. Needless to say this is discouraging."

"My daughter, eleven years old, is about 75 pounds overweight. She is considered a 'slow child' and food has become an obsession with her. . . . I know nagging her and belittling her are not the answer. . . . The children's doctor's only help has been handing us a diet and telling us to keep rich food out of the house. It hasn't helped."

"I have been overweight thirty-one years (all of my life) and never married due to a feeling of fat inferiority. I'm desperate!"

"I do not have trouble losing weight, but rather in keeping it off. I have not yet established in my mind where to draw the line and how to teach myself that it comes right back on even easier if you don't watch yourself. . . . My boyfriend and I plan to get married toward the end of this year and I do want to look extravagant in my wedding gown—and super for the honeymoon. He also wants me to lose it before he will marry me. When we first met I was 123 pounds and today I am 168 pounds—big difference."

"I have just recently lost weight, thinking that

was going to be the hardest part, but the hardest part for me is now resisting overly indulging myself in food as I have previously."

"As a moderately successful Weight Watcher I find the energy I expend just staying 'legal' is exhausting and causes more stress for me. I realize the weight problem is a matter of mental attitude but I haven't found the 'tools' or the direction I need to conquer this nightmare of living in a fat body."

"I am only twenty-four years old; however, I have been dieting (mostly unsuccessfully) for about ten years. The struggle, I have come to realize, is the state of one's mind. I believe almost any diet can be successful if one can approach it from a proper frame of mind. Although my weight is not that out of hand (about 20 pounds), to me it has always been monumental. The conflict arises out of my disgust with being constantly overweight and yet never achieving a positive attitude toward losing weight."

"I'm very scared of my weight, and desperately would like to lose 30 or 35 pounds. Is this possible? I've tried many diets and can't stick to them."

"I have a son twenty-one years old who weighs 450 pounds. No doctor that we have taken him to seems to want to do anything but put him on a diet. I think he needs more help than that."

"I'm fat—320 pounds—sickening, isn't it? I've tried all kinds of diets . . . but they've all failed—or I failed them. I'm only twenty-three and I'm sick of myself. So sick I sometimes don't care if I continue to live. Yet, I find myself eating, eating, eating . . ."

"I am sixty-three years old, and have had a weight problem for as long as I can remember. . . . I am grossly obese. I fear for my life. I know these extra pounds will rob me of years of life—probably already have—and I have much to live for. I lost 30 pounds on an 800-calorie diet, but have gained it all back since reverting to bad eating habits."

"I know that I need to work on my head in order to remove the 30 pounds that I put on three years ago during a period of stress. I have been unable to cut down my food for any sustained period of time; I need help to break the cycle of self-hate and despair over my present physical appearance especially."

"I have used some of your ideas to stop smoking. However, one can give up cigarettes because they can be avoided, but we cannot avoid food. It is needed to sustain life, and once my mouth is open it never stops."

"It's great knowing that my fantasies can be put to good use for me. You have relieved me of the conviction that to daydream is a waste of time. You have proven it is not. You offer a positive cheap way to gain control of your problems without the use of drugs. Your mind trips are a marvelous way to become thin while relieving the stress which created the problem."

Overweight people do not need disapproval, moral judgments, crash diets, or admonitions to "stop eating so much." That is no more effective than telling an alcoholic to cut down on his drinking. They need help in learning to control overeating.

You need to know how *to stop overeating.*

A major reason diets fail ultimately is that after you reach your desired weight you don't have any more self-rewards to keep your weight steady. As the behavioral psychologists have found out, people can be motivated, as can rats in cages, by rewards and punishments. And there is nothing wrong with that. Most successful people reward themselves constantly, and so, incidentally, do most people who lose weight successfully.

Now, psychologically, what happens when you are on an ordinary diet plan? You exert tremendous "will power," you lose weight, and the rewards you get are from seeing the scales go down, your clothes become loose, and your friends and family comment on your progress. For a while these—especially the proof on the scale—can be powerful. Like a laboratory rat, you have been doing something effective to earn your reward. And you feel good about it, which reinforces it. But suppose the trainer stops showing up with the cheese, or the electrical stimulations to the pleasure centers of the brain? The incentive disappears. This happens when you lose as many or nearly as many pounds as you want. You no longer have the feedback from the scales, friends become nonchalant about your new appearance, and you gradually "fall off the wagon." And the vicious cycle of regaining begins again.

The problem is that the self-reward spurring you onward to exert your will power has been the actual losing of the weight. When this discontinues, you are bereft, because you do not have sufficient other self-rewards to keep you going. You have not learned them. The best kinds of self-rewards are internal, but we have found, as have other researchers, that overweight people often make less effective use of psychic self-rewards than thin people. (And unfortunately, a lot of overweight people have learned to reward themselves with food, which is counterproductive, to say the least.) After you lose weight, the immediate reinforcement needed to keep up the diet vanishes.

Another drawback of the conventional diet is

that the body doesn't lose weight consistently, even when you eat fewer calories consistently. There are ups and downs. Especially in the beginning of a diet, you may be encouraged by enormous weight loss, which, in fact, is fluid. Often when people who stay on calorie-restricted diets don't lose weight steadily (as monitored daily by their scales) they become disillusioned; they think their diet isn't working—that is, their reward is not forthcoming—so they junk the diet and start overeating again.

Weight loss, on its own, is not an immediate or long-lasting enough reward to be effective for most people.

To lose weight successfully, you must reward yourself for the *actions* that caused you to lose weight, and not just for the weight loss itself. After a while these acts will be ingrained in your mind, become habits, and take over automatically. Studies repeatedly show that you lose weight more successfully if you tie your self-rewards to changing habits and thinking than to anything else.

12

EATING BY THE CLOCK

Why do you eat too much? The reasons may be numerous, but it is almost certainly not because you are physically hungry. One might think hunger is a universal phenomenon keyed directly to man's primitive needs. But it isn't. The nourishment many of us seek from food is not physical but psychological. In fact, our hunger mechanisms have become so distorted that most of us have never experienced true hunger, do not recognize it, and do not use it as a triggering device for eating. Nor do we know when we are full, or use fullness as a signal to stop eating.

We're more likely to be driven to eat by a "mouth hunger" or a "desire to eat" (controlled by the mind, we may add), which has little or nothing to do with stomach pangs.

When Albert J. Stunkard, at the University of

Pennsylvania, monitored the stomach contractions of two groups—one obese, one normal-weighted—he found that the overeaters simply could not judge when they were physically hungry. They often said they felt hungry when their stomachs showed no contractions that would indicate physical hunger. It's also been shown that problem eaters will often eat as much on a full stomach as on an empty one, and sometimes more. On the other hand, people without weight problems tend to hear and listen to hunger pains. They generally don't overeat when they are full, and Stunkard found that their reports of hunger corresponded pretty well with their stomach contractions.

Thus, overeating is usually switched on and off not by physical mechanisms but by psychic ones. Eating, in fact, for many, is a ritual with emotionally charged overtones. In hospital settings where food and surroundings are drab, overweight people often automatically cut their calorie consumption from over 3,000 daily to 500, whereas normal-weighted patients consume about the same daily number of calories as usual.

Overeaters are also likely to be stimulated to eat by the mere sight of food. If you see it, you want it. If it's out of sight, you may not think about it, or make much effort to get it. You may even totally forget about it until you lay eyes on it; then it seems irresistible.

Especially interesting is that many people literally eat by the clock, even if the clock is wrong. Researchers Stanley Schachter and Larry Gross, also at the University of Pennsylvania, tinkered with two clocks so that one ran at half normal speed and the other at twice normal speed. On the pretense of being given a "personality" test, obese (defined as 14 to 75 percent overweight by national charts) and normal subjects were left in a room with one or the other of the clocks—and a box of crackers. By the time a true half-hour had passed, one clock would read 5:20, and the other 6:05. As you may have guessed, it made little difference what time the clock read for the normal-weighted. In fact, the closer it got to their dinner hour, the less they ate, because they didn't want to spoil their dinners. On the other hand, the overweight responded by eating twice as much when the clock said 6:05 as when it said 5:20. In short, the clock, faulty as it was, told them to eat and they did.

Emotional upsets of any kind will often trigger overeating. Many people substitute food for direct ways of dealing with emotional upsets. They literally "swallow" their anger or nibble away out of anxiety or boredom. Overweight people will even eat more when frightened; thinner people often eat less at times of intense fear.

Since people who overeat are usually eating for sheer pleasure instead of nourishment, they are often attracted by good-tasting food. Still, they usually don't get as much pleasure from each bite as they should, because they don't take time to taste the food. Numerous findings, including ours, indicate that in general, people with weight problems eat faster than thinner ones, chewing less, savoring less. Some bolt down food, as one said, "like a wolf." In truth, many overeaters eat without thinking or tasting.

13

POOH'S INSIGHT

Remember A.A. Milne's *The House at Pooh Corner?*

"What do you like best in the world, Pooh?"

"Well," said Pooh, "what I like best"—and then he had to stop and think.

Because although eating honey *was* a very good thing to do, there was a moment just before you began to eat it which was better than when you were, but he didn't know what it was called.

If we may supply the word for Pooh, it is "anticipation," and it is merely a kind of imagination.

Part of your "mouth hunger" is formed by an old image in your mind of how a certain food will taste. At one time, perhaps as a child, you may have really enjoyed that food. But if you stopped to really taste

it today, you might find it unappealing. The image of
the food may exert far more power than the actual
eating.

In our program we have people take a test
adapted from one developed by the psychologist
Frank J. Bruno. They put a favorite food in front of
them, and observe it steadily for five minutes; they
intensively study its texture, contemplate its color,
and imagine how it will taste. If at the end of the five
minutes they still want to eat it, they can. Some do,
and some don't—it doesn't make any difference in
the success of doing the exercise. But, after intensively studying the food, some become turned off,
and have no desire to eat it. They see that the old
photograph in their mind does not coincide with the
food in real life. In some instances the mind picture
changes so the food becomes downright objectionable. For example, one man began to view his melt-
ing ice cream as sperm. A woman who examined her
favorite caramel-covered marshmallow, cut in half,
began to see it as a piece of cotton.

Those who do eat it often confess that it did not
meet expectations. As a result of this exercise, the
mind picture begins to change to conform to reality,
and certain foods people have overdosed on for years
turn them off. Many find it unbelievable; they take a
bite, then refuse to eat any more because it doesn't
"taste good."

We also have people, while blindfolded, taste
small pieces of a variety of foods: cooked potato,
sweet onion, mild cheese, cake, and so on. When not
told what they are tasting, they can't tell much difference. Says one: "Onion tasted just like potato to me."
Without the visual trappings, it is true, you often
can't tell which food is which. It is the visual come-

on, which food advertisers fully exploit, that is often the trap. When you discover food often doesn't really taste as good as your image says it should, you have come far in breaking its hold on you.

The most crucial fact from all such observations and studies is that your overeating may be triggered, not by *internal* physical events, but by *external* events, of which you are unaware and over which you seemingly have little control. It is this lack of internal control that makes eating seem frightening to some. A thin person, guided by an internal self-adjusting mechanism, can go on an occasional binge without anxiety, because he knows in his mind he has total control over the eating situation. Such a person always can accept or reject food next time without anxiety. But if you don't know what is driving you to eat, you may feel that your fate is in the hands of mysterious forces you don't know how to control. (Yet you may do perfectly well in other areas of your life. Many people we see are quite successful in their jobs, for example: they are business executives, authors, management consultants, lawyers, physicians, even psychologists. In this one area of overeating they have not learned the same kind of inner control that has made them successful elsewhere.)

There's no doubt many of us, even those mildly overweight, have learned to respond to food as if we were laboratory rats chasing a piece of cheese. When the bell rings inside our heads, we want it. We don't know why we want it—we just want it.

The problem is not in the stomach, but in the mind.

Eating for many people who want to lose weight is thus triggered by outside stimuli. Some people eat the minute they walk in the door at home, the instant they see the refrigerator, the minute the TV set is switched on, when they go to a party, visit their mother, turn on music, start to read, feel anxious or bored, get angry, feel depressed or have an argument, feel overworked. They are seized by the desire to eat. Yet, many don't make the connections between the "stimulus" that caused them to run for the food and their overeating. However, somewhere in your mind, you know what that stimulus is, and you can discover it, if you let yourself, and destroy its power to affect your eating.

14

CHANGING PATTERNS

Losing weight is a *learning* process, or a relearning process, in which, slowly but surely, your attitudes and responses toward food change. The accumulation of old directives in your mind crumbles, and they are replaced by new directives which tend to become a permanent part of your self. Once the new attitudes and responses are assimilated, you would have to go through the same procedure in reverse to change them back. Thus you effect a change, a true change inside your head. It involves modifying your self-image and your notions of "success and failure," and the things that trigger you to eat.

The process is not negative; it is entirely positive. People emerge with stronger, more assertive, positive feelings about themselves. They learn to find joy in other things besides eating. They begin to see themselves as the persons they knew they could be. Mainly, they develop a marvelous control over their eating that boosts feelings of competence, power, and self-esteem.

You have the resources inside you to do this; you are the person responsible. Your fate is not regulated by forces beyond your control. Almost everything you now do comes from repetition of long-forgotten patterns. If you learned them once, you can unlearn them now, replacing them with new thin-producing patterns.

Consistent with this:

1. Weight loss should be *gradual* and steady, the consequences of your *changing eating patterns,* and not of a crash diet. Every pound lost then becomes representative not of some abnormal exertion of will power, but of actual inner control. Further, with every performance, the new pattern is strengthened, ensuring its continuance. This makes it a lasting victory. Remember, this is all about changing internally —not losing weight. The by-product is losing weight for good.

Losing 2 pounds a week is excellent, if it does not reappear. Losing 10 pounds this week is an insignificant victory—in fact, it is a defeat—if it is back in three months, or sooner. Because weight loss itself is not the criterion of a success, we advise people not to weigh themselves once a day. Do it only once a week at the same time with shoes off. Then record your weight on a chart. You can then take pride in the weight curve going downward. But a plateau should not be disturbing. If you are practicing the mind trips and absorbing new mind patterns, your weight will go down, sometimes more quickly than you expect.

2. *Restrictive* dieting is counterproductive. We do not encourage going on a rigid diet, though we do, of course, think it essential to cut down on calorie consumption as a result of better eating habits. Sometimes physicians we work with provide calorie limits for their patients. We also think a good calorie counter necessary to correct faulty thinking. For we discover that some people have no realistic concept of how many calories a food contains. Men especially are often convinced beef is low in calories. When they realize this is not true, they are often happy to switch to chicken or fish, which are much less fattening. On the other hand, many mistakenly believe potatoes, spaghetti, and bread are outrageously fattening, when they are not. Others tend to underestimate the high calorie counts of sweets, mainly pies and cakes.

We do not say you cannot eat these things; we only ask you to be aware of how many calories you are consuming by eating them. We also in the beginning ask people for the first week or so to keep a daily food sheet, noting what they eat, when they eat it, and how many calories it contains. Without such a record, most people have little idea what they are eating and when. Just being aware usually produces a cut in calories.

If there are a few foods you find particularly devastating, you may want to give them up temporarily, or at least cut down on their consumption. But it is detrimental to play the self-denial game of constructing a long list of forbidden foods. It is our credo that you can eat *anything* as long as you don't overdo it. Two tablespoons of any food can give sufficient satisfaction. Dr. Stern, for

example, keeps three boxes of her favorite choco-
lates in a drawer. She eats one or two pieces a
day. If you are saying to yourself, "I can't do that,"
you are wrong. You can do it.

You, not the food, are in control.

15

WHY MIND TRIPS

Unfortunately, weight loss is usually attacked as if it had little to do with psychological factors. Or when it is approached from a psychological perspective, the program is usually very narrow, consisting of habit-breaking techniques. That is not enough. Losing weight is hardly an isolated problem. It involves complex personal dynamics. It may involve restructuring your thinking, wiping out irrational or erroneous concepts, modifying the silent statements and instructions you give yourself. It may involve digging up, examining, and confronting old childhood patterns of eating, or becoming aware of the emotional obstacles to losing weight. It may involve finding ways to vent feelings that do not lead to overeating. It may involve finding alternatives to eating, and learning how to reward yourself and make yourself feel good.

In short, permanent weight control demands a comprehensive mind change. Such a program is used at our institute, and the results have been phenomenal. Over 70 percent of our clients have lost significant amounts of weight—four have lost as much as 64 pounds in a 14-week period—and 75 percent of them have not regained their weight in a year's time. Our latest research shows that those in our program who used imagery extensively lost an average of 21 pounds. In comparison, a control group not in our program who used no imagery and relied on fasting, weight clubs and drugs, lost only an average of one pound in the same amount of time. These figures are remarkable compared with the failure rate of other weight-loss regimens.

We have long used mind trips in our weight-loss program. But we are increasingly using them because of their astounding potency in promoting mind change. Thus, we have devised mind trips to incorporate all of the concepts that have produced such success among our clients. You will find these trips in this book. They are carefully constructed to produce the same kind of success that our clients have experienced.

The secret of the mind trips is that they greatly accelerate mind change and are incredibly efficient in instilling new eating patterns. Meticulously designed, they can transport you to a state of mind where change takes place more easily and sometimes instantly.

Assuming there was enough time, all of us could probably be conditioned like rats in a laboratory to change our habits. But, because we are humans, what is necessary for animals is not necessary for us. We have the resource, our imagery, to learn directly, each one of us, *inside* our heads. Assuming a person had adequate physical coordination, he or she could practice and become a passable golfer, tennis player, or even pianist. But what a shortcut we have when we can do much of the practicing in our heads through imagery, as experiments prove. Given enough therapeutic sessions, most of us could, if we wanted, alter our lives. But how much more quickly we can do it through guided daydreams, as shown by European therapists. If we have an irrational fear, we might eventually conquer it with "talk therapy." But what a model of efficiency is Wolpe's imagery trips for phobic desensitization.

The same thing is true in weight control. People can search their minds consciously for what makes them eat. Often, after trial and error, they come up with what they believe is the right answer. But the mind trips which reveal the same answer in instantaneous communication are much faster. Through imagery, you may discover instantly what can take frustrating weeks to discover by keeping charts and paying close attention to eating. This indeed does happen, and people are totally amazed. They know the answers that surface are true. There is no need for further guesswork about the nature of your eating problems once the mind has spoken. The mind does not lie; it represents your truest self and guides your actions.

Everything you need to lose weight is inside your head.

The mind trips can reveal to you the true reason for your eating. They can also help you discover and symbolically overcome obstacles to losing weight, paving the way to actual control of eating; help you rehearse eating habits that will cause you to lose weight; allow you to test out new ways of eating without dire consequences; help instill an inner self-control; help you relax and "get away from it all"; teach you to deal with difficult eating situations; act as self-rewards; and promote a sense of well-being.

The mind trips have any number of pluses. You need no elaborate equipment, as you do in bio-feedback, for example. There are no side effects, as there may be with drugs. They are simple to learn; they require no special training or education. They are easy to perform and take little time—only about ten minutes a day. You don't have to go anywhere outside the house or to a special place to use them. They are suitable for routine use, and if you miss a day, their effectiveness is not lost. Probably the most miraculous aspect of the mind trips, which makes them so effective, is that they allow you to interject into the process your own self with your unique eating problems and your own unique potential for solving them.

Most important, you get *immediate* and *continuous* results, and spin-offs in other areas of your life. Most who have used mind trips are happier, more assertive, and more confident people as well as *thinner* people. And they stay that way.

PART THREE

The Mind Trips

16

HOW TO DO MIND TRIPS

Before you start to use the mind trips, here are some things we want you to know:

Anyone can use the mind trips. You do not have to have any special talent for imaging, though it is true that the more vividly you experience the trips, the more value they will have. When we ask you to image something, we want you to call into your mind's eye an imagined scene or event as vividly as you can. Experience it as much as possible, as if you were living or reliving it. Become a part of it. Try to see the shapes and the colors, and experience the smells, sounds, and most important your own emotions at what you are "seeing."

However, visualizing in your inner self is not quite the same as seeing something with your eyes, so don't be discouraged or disappointed if the image doesn't come as clearly to you as in a photograph. The way you visualize is the way you visualize, and the more you do it, the better you will be able to do it.

The mind trips, as you will see, are carefully constructed to guide your mind for the best results. However, they are not so constricting as to include every last detail; that would preclude your own self from entering the picture fully with your own interpretations and experience. In some cases, as with Jungle Doors, you are asked to open a door in your mind so that an image can spontaneously pop into it. Some of the images that appear during the mind trips may be disturbing. If so, you can stop the trip by saying, "STOP," or you can face it squarely (in the case of Jungle Doors, you can slam the door on the image)—whichever you are ready to do. Nevertheless, though an image is disturbing, it has significance for you, and it has now come into your awareness, where you can deal with it if you choose to; it no longer remains hidden and beyond your control. Thus, there is a positive benefit to some amounts of anxiety.

There is no *wrong* way of doing the trips. Sometimes in our sessions people will say, "I know I am doing it wrong," merely because they found that someone else did it another way. In one case, when asked to visualize a rock, a woman explained she had chosen one that used to be in her back yard as a child. She asked, "Wasn't that wrong? Because I simply remembered it?" She felt it had to be some fictional rock that she completely "made up." Since everything that comes into your mind as an image fragment has been placed there consciously or subliminally by your memory, it is impossible to have one image "real" and another fictional. Your images are the sum total of your experience, and what we are asking is for you to experience your own images, whatever they are.

Further, do not try to force the images. They will come into your mind regardless and without effort. And accept those that do come into your mind— don't reject them as absurd or invalid. They are valid for you.

Some people have asked the question, "If I go into my mind, won't I stay there? Won't I lose touch with reality?" As you will quickly see, you never lose touch with what's going on around you. You do not go into what could be called a hypnotic trance. You enter what we call another level of reality, but it does not preclude your participating in what we ordinarily call the real world. While you are doing the meta-images you will be perfectly aware and able to respond if the phone rings or a child calls. You are conscious. It is much like driving a car. Once you learn to drive, you don't have to pay conscious attention to every movement of your arm, foot, or eyes, yet if something unexpected comes up, your attention is instantly available.

Before taking each mind trip, read it through carefully. Then get comfortable, either lying down or sitting up. You can preface each trip with one of the relaxation exercises given here, or take a deep breath and hold it for seven seconds until you are relaxed. We have found, as have other researchers, that relaxation is a good prelude for getting you into the mind trips.

Close your eyes. Though it's possible for some people to do the trips with eyes open, for most people closing the eyes is much preferred, for it shuts out external disruptions that demand your conscious attention. With eyes closed you can better focus on your inner self where the mind trips will take place.

Each mind trip is designed to meet a special purpose which we have found valuable in controlling weight. Some of them will undoubtedly be more effective for you than others. We suggest that you try the ones you think you would like and repeat those which seem to have the most meaning for you. Repetition of some of the trips is essential for completing the mind change, and these we will point out to you.

If there are some trips you don't want to try, don't. Some people are reluctant to try the "aversive" trips, even though they have proved powerful. Which trips you take is up to you. We suggest, however, that you choose the ones that do you the most good, and do them for ten minutes a day. You may be surprised how quickly you notice results. Many report immediate insights that alter their eating habits.

While doing the trips, take your time, giving yourself enough time to experience them fully. If you want, you can have someone read the trips to you, pausing several seconds between instructions to give you time enough to complete them. You could also read the trips yourself into a tape recorder, and follow the instructions when each is played back. Dr. Stern has put many of the trips on tapes, which are available through the Institute for Behavioral Awareness.

Since some of the mind trips will reveal surprises and insights to you, you may want to think more about what appeared to you in the images. Often you can gain further awareness by talking about your experience with someone who knows you well, such as your spouse or a good friend. It's not only fun to share your experience, but by so doing, you often get more benefit by receiving feedback or additional information from someone else.

Don't be bothered if for some reason some of the mind trips in which you are directed to image yourself don't give you a complete picture of yourself. When we ask our clients what they like best about themselves, most invariably say their heads, fingernails, and toes. When you are overweight your body is often something you don't want to face—realistically —so you may resist producing a true image of yourself in your mind. That doesn't matter. Flow with the mind trips, as they present themselves to you. As you change, so will your ability to accept yourself.

For example, one of our teenage girls had set as a goal the purchase of a bikini. She used the Staircase mind trip to get the experience of how great she would feel when she was thin enough to wear the bikini. Her staircase was carpeted in red, much like the one in the movie *Gone with the Wind,* and at the top she could see this image of a person in a bikini; she knew it was herself, and she experienced the thrill of knowing how good she felt standing there in the bikini. But she could not bring herself to image her own body; she could see her own head; but the body she imaged was always that of a thinner friend. Then, when the time for her to get the bikini was only two weeks away, as she was doing the mind trip one day, it was no longer her friend she saw standing in the bikini. She saw herself. It was a major victory. As her self-concept changed, she had come to accept it and be able to picture it. We have seen such remarkable changes dozens of times. They are the norm, rather than the exception.

17

BASIC MIND TRIPS

PRACTICE

Before you begin, if you have any doubts about your ability to form mental pictures, you might want to try these simple exercises. They demonstrate how easy it is.

Rock: Look down at your lap. A rock is resting there. How large is it? What is the color and shape of the rock? "Touch" your rock. What does it feel like? Is it smooth or rough, cool or warm to the touch? Fill in all the characteristics of this particular rock. Is it a rock you have seen before or a new one you made up? Now pick up your rock and throw it. Pick it up again and throw it somewhere else.

Ping-Pong: Close your eyes and picture a Ping-Pong game. The day is warm and you are sitting under the sun. The slight breeze feels good as it passes across your body and ruffles your hair. The players are dressed in white, facing each other across the Ping-Pong table, which is green and marked off with white lines. Now watch the game progress. The first player hits the ball to his opponent, who returns it easily. The ball goes back and forth. Watch it until one player does not hit the ball back.

Eating an Orange: Close your eyes. You are sitting at a table with a plate in front of you. An orange is on the plate. Look at the skin and the color of the orange. Pick it up and cut it into four segments. Watch the juice flow from it. See the seeds, white membrane, and pulp. Pick up a segment and bring it toward your nose. Smell it. Now slowly begin to eat the orange segment.

If you are like most people who try this exercise, you will begin to salivate even before you have "eaten" the orange.

BODY RELAXATION

Sometimes you may be so tense that you cannot get into the imagery. If so, here is a body-relaxation exercise you can use to relax. It is adapted from one used at the New Jersey Neuro-Psychiatric Institute in Princeton. Eventually, if you practice enough, you will only need to take a deep breath (as in the last part of the exercise) to become fully relaxed. Sometimes, just being relaxed will guide you away from overeating.

Sit or lie in a comfortable position. Close your

eyes. Raise your hands and make a fist. Tighten them. Feel the tightness across your knuckles. Tighten your wrists. Tense each forearm and now your elbows. Zero in on the tight feeling. Now tense each upper arm. Make each entire hand and arm tighter and tighter until it trembles. Concentrate on feeling the muscles involved; sense them becoming as taut as wound up springs. Hold it for seven seconds. Now just drop your arms. Go with the good feeling as the spring unwinds. Experience the feeling of relaxation that comes with it. Feel calm and comfortable. Relaxed, just relaxed and wonderfully, wonderfully well.

Now make a face; frown and tense the muscles around your mouth and around your eyes. Feel the muscles tighten across your cheeks and lips. Feel your jaw muscles tighten. Wrinkle your nose. Tighten the muscles in your chin. Now tighten your forehead. Hold it for about seven seconds. Experience the tensions as the muscles all over your face become tighter and tighter. Now relax your face. Let all of your facial muscles go. Experience the feeling as your mouth relaxes, your eyes relax, and your cheeks and jaw loosen up. Feel your lips and chin relax, and the muscles in your forehead. Go with the good, comfortable feeling. Feel fine, good, and wonderfully, wonderfully well, calm, and relaxed.

Arch your back and raise up your chest. Hold it. Experience the pull as the muscles between your shoulder blades become taut, and hold it for seven seconds. Now relax. Allow your back and chest to drop. Experience the wonderful, soothing feeling as you do so. Feel comfortable and relaxed.

Now pull in your stomach and abdomen. Tighten your stomach and make it as hard as a rock —harder—harder. Feel the tension in your stomach.

Experience the muscles in your abdomen tighten. Hold it, again for seven seconds. Now just let go. Sink back and relax. Experience the wonderful feeling of relaxation throughout your stomach. Feel the abdominal muscles go gentle, feel totally relaxed and comfortable, and just great.

Stretch out your legs. Tighten the muscles in your thighs. Feel your thighs getting tighter and tighter like a tightly wound rubber band. Now also tighten the muscles in your knees; feel them tense up. Tighten the muscles in your calves. Turn your toes under and tighten each entire foot. Experience the tightness up and down each leg, in your ankle and your toes. Make each leg tighter, tighter, and hold it for seven seconds.

Now let go; just drop your legs and experience the wonderful sensation as the muscles in each leg relax. Feel your thighs, your knees, your calves, your ankles relax. Feel the restful feeling as even your toes go limp. Notice how good it feels to unwind . . . from head to toe.

Now take a deep breath and concentrate on the air filling your lungs. Hold it for seven seconds or so. Now let go, let out your breath and feel the wonderful sensation as your tensions and worries slowly, slowly disappear as they go out of you with your breath. You are feeling relaxed, peaceful, and comfortable, wonderfully, wonderfully well.

Remember to do this sequence as many times as needed to feel deeply, comfortably relaxed.

FAVORITE PLACE

Everyone should have a place to escape to where they feel relaxed, comfortable, at peace. And you can create such a haven in your head. You can then use such a mental picture in many constructive ways: to relax, to counter negative feelings, as a self-reward, as a means of boosting your spirits.

In some of the upcoming trips, you will be instructed to counteract a negative or aversive image with a positive one, and the "favorite place" trip is an ideal one to use. It is important to develop the mind trip so that you can have it instantly available when you need it and do not have to go searching around your mind, wondering where you could find peace at that moment.

To develop the meta-image, simply close your eyes and picture yourself in a place where you are at perfect peace. Be there alone. If there are other people, let them be strangers in crowds, apart from you. Develop the scene in all its details. Put yourself into the picture. Experience all of it. Many people choose a beach, or a place they once vacationed. It doesn't matter whether it is a place you have once been or a fantasy place you "made up." It is only important that it be a place you feel you would like to be at any time—your favorite place.

18

IDENTIFYING YOUR PROBLEMS

EATING DRAMA

Purpose: To help you assess your eating situation. Often we find that a person's eating history and current situation are like a theatrical event, with highs, lows, dialogue, a theme, and often an ending.

❧

Picture a TV or movie screen. You are going to play out your Eating Drama on the screen. The music starts and the screen credits come on. The title, "My Eating Drama" by (your name), flashes across the screen. You will see your eating behavior shown on the screen. You will see your successes and your failures. You will note your feelings. Who else is involved in your eating drama? Watch it from beginning to end. Take your time. Is this show a comedy, a tragedy, a soap opera, a farce, or a mixture of these things? Image an audience watching this show. What do they do? Do they applaud, cry, boo, laugh, go to sleep, or demand their money back? Do you agree with them?

❧❦

This trip is like a diagnosis. It gives you a chance to take a total look at the "life script" you have written for yourself concerning eating. If, after doing the trip, you take time to analyze it, you will get more out of it.

Can you detect a general theme? Some psychological feeling that permeates the entire production? Even the kind of music in your drama offers a clue to your theme. Some people hear sad, melodramatic music; others, especially fast eaters, hear the frenetic piano-pounding of the 1920s Mack Sennett silent films. Some hear no music at all. Many people in our program are startled to realize that their eating dramas resolve around failure and personal helplessness, or resentment and anger turned inward. Some common themes are: "I can't help it." "You made me do it." "Poor little me." "It's not my fault." Some are also astounded to hear the negative dialogue coming from themselves and other actors. For others the theme is a desire for security or love.

It is interesting also to explore the audience reactions. Did they get your message? Is it a message you want people to get about you? Is this the message you are also giving inwardly to yourself?

You'll undoubtedly derive some fascinating insights from this trip. It will give you a general awareness of your eating situation, opening the way for change.

JUNGLE DOORS

Purpose: To help you discover hidden psychological obstacles that are blocking your progress in losing weight. Once you bring the barriers into your awareness, you can begin to devise effective ways to deal with them. Also, the trip helps you exercise some immediate symbolic control over the obstacles by telling yourself they are not going to stop you, or by slamming the door on them.

❧

Picture yourself in a dense jungle. You are walking along a narrow path, slowly and carefully. Look at the strange flowers, listen to the strange sounds of birds and animals. Notice the unusual plants and trees, and feel the grasses brush against your legs as you walk. The jungle smells musty and you catch a whiff of some exotic flower's perfume. As you walk, you come upon a door. You know that behind that door is a stumbling block—something that gets in the way of healthy, appropriate eating and losing weight. Something that acts as a barrier to your being more successful at permanent weight control. It is something that gets in your way, something quite specific.

Now open the door, and look at what is there. Experience whatever is behind the door. Notice it thoroughly. Study it. Become completely involved in what is behind the door that is getting in your way.

Now, say to yourself: "This is not going to stop me from being successful. I will not allow this to get

in my way anymore!" Slam the door and walk away.
Continue through the jungle, and open and close as
many other doors as you wish. Then when you are
finished, walk quickly out of the jungle, where you
will find a beach. Relax for a while on the beach.

This trip is guaranteed to turn up some surprises.
Many people are startled at what they find behind
the doors; nevertheless they often instantly recognize the obstacles as true ones of which they have
been consciously unaware.

For example, every time one woman in our program lost 10 pounds or so her husband would bring
her a surprise cake or candy, which she would eat
because she didn't want to hurt his feelings. When
she opened her Jungle Door she found her husband
standing there smiling. Though she had long vaguely
sensed he was somehow consciously or unconsciously
sabotaging her weight-loss efforts, she had never
seen it clearly enough to resist. Once she did acknowledge what was happening, she started discouraging him, then worked up courage to ask him
not to bring the food and to give her more support.
He did.

In another instance, a woman discovered nothing more profound behind the Jungle Door than the
back door to her house. She was puzzled until she
realized she always came home from work through
the back door, which led directly into the kitchen;
this set off an impulse to eat. Her simple solution,
which worked, was to go around and come in the
front door, avoiding temptation.

Thus, what you may find is anything from the

most obvious mundane stumbling blocks, which are easy to rectify, to the most intensely personal ones. You never know which it is going to be. The important point is that once you are aware of the obstacles, you can think up constructive ways to deal with them. As long as they remain hidden there is little hope of conquering them.

This is one trip you will want to do over and over, for different obstacles show up depending on current circumstances. It is rare that one obstacle pops up over and over. Clearing up one problem, therefore, may not solve all your weight problems. Other obstacles may also be there, waiting to appear. The more of them you discover and clear up, the better your chances of achieving permanent weight loss.

MOUNTAIN CLIMBING

Purpose: This trip is designed to give you much information about what may be standing in your way of reaching the top of the "mountain," that is, lasting weight loss. It also helps you get "unstuck" in your efforts by letting you devise imaginative ways to overcome the obstacles. If you can symbolically remove the obstacles during the mountain climb, your chances of doing the same for weight control in real life are increased.

Picture a small mountain or hill that goes up, but not too sharply. Picture the whole scene. Notice what kind of day it is. Is it winter or summer? Notice what you are wearing. Look at the top of the mountain. Feel how you want to get to the top and enjoy the view. You want to be successful in losing weight.

You begin to move up the path toward the top of the mountain. As you walk, you find the path strewn with small rocks—obstacles to permanently losing weight. Kick them aside and continue on your way. As you wind around and up, you find that the obstacles are getting larger. Notice what the obstacles are in detail. Then remove each one in any way you can. Continue going upward until you run into an obstacle that won't budge. It is too large or too deeply embedded in the earth for you to remove it. Look at the situation the obstacle represents. Try to think of a way to get past it. Can you climb over it? Go around it? Get someone to help you remove it? Can you squeeze by?

When you get past, you find you are at the top of the mountain. You feel a little tired, but exhilarated. Give yourself time to look at and enjoy the view.

For some the journey is a struggle, and not everyone manages to get to the top on the first try. However, as you practice and progress in learning new habits for losing weight, your ability to detect and overcome specific eating problems drastically increases. Some people, freed by imagery, devise imaginative ways to get rid of the stubborn roadblock in their way. Some have used a raygun to break it up, a crane to carry it off. Some have stared it out of existence. Some have actually devoured it. Some people's boulders have grown feet and walked away.

After doing the trip, try to analyze what you

learned during the mountain climbing. What were the obstacles? Did they involve you or other people? Did they involve eating times, such as after dinner, or situations, such as bingeing? Or eating too much food or the wrong kind—for example, junk food that doesn't satisfy? Think also about how you removed the obstacles. Can you think of any way to do that in real life? Consider what the positive payoff would be if you did remove the obstacles.

DOUBLE CHAIRS

Purpose: This meta-image is adapted from a technique used extensively by the psychologist Fritz Perls. Perls believed you could work through conflicting feelings by creating a dialogue with yourself as you shifted back and forth between two chairs. That way, you can present both sides of a conflict and perhaps integrate them into a solution. You can use this trip to work through many conflicts that revolve around food.

Picture yourself in a room that has two chairs that face each other. Image all the other details in the room. Is it a comfortable room, one you like? The chairs look comfortable. What color are they? Are they made of metal or wood, or are they upholstered? Sit down in one of these chairs, facing the other one. Relax and get comfortable. Begin talking to the opposite chair. State one side of the conflict. Explain the situation, what the problem is, and how you feel about it. Now mentally switch chairs. Image getting up and crossing over to the other chair. You are now ready to answer the first chair. Explain the opposing side of the conflict. Try to answer as truthfully as you can. When you have finished, once again move from the second chair back to the first chair again, and answer from that point of view. Continue to change chairs until you have examined both sides of the question thoroughly and come to some decision about the conflicting situation.

After the trip, take a few minutes to reflect on what happened. How do you feel about it? Did any surprising hidden feelings show up? If you made a decision as a result of the dialogue, do you think it will help you lose weight? If so, how? To make sure you focus on problem-solving, you might regard one chair as the "problem presenter" and the other chair as the "problem solver." This double-chair dialogue will help you work out current conflicts surrounding food when you aren't sure what you really want to do.

EMOTIONAL CLOSET

Purpose: You undoubtedly have certain feelings about food which you have had since childhood. These feelings are not necessarily deep and dark, but like other feelings they are probably so diffuse you can't quite put your finger on them. They are still hidden behind "closed doors"—beyond your conscious vision.

In this trip, you open the door to recognize and confront old feelings about food that may no longer be appropriate. The purpose is to notice not only *what* you see, but *how you feel* about what you see. By bringing the feelings into the open, you can begin to deal with them or just allow them to exist.

☙❧

You are going on a tour through a house or an apartment. You are at the front door. Open it. Feel the weight of the door and your hand on the handle as you turn it. Walk inside and close the door behind you. Image the room you are now in. Look at the furniture, the colors of the walls, the shape of things. Allow yourself to fully experience being in this room.

Now, move on into the next room. What kind of room is it? What is it used for? Allow yourself to experience standing in this room, being in it and looking around. Now move into another room, a room that has a closet in it. Think of the total room. What kind of room is it? What is it used for? Now turn your attention to the closet in this room. As you approach the closet you experience a vague familiar sensation, a *déjà vu* feeling that you have been here before and that there are things in this particular closet that belong to you. You realize that this is an "emotional closet" and behind its door you have stored up and saved all your ideas and feelings about food, about eating and overeating. Now open the door and look in. Experience what you find in the closet. Try to experience all of it as fully as possible. Become aware of your feelings as you handle the fears, memories, people, good things and bad. When you have gone through all of the things in your emotional closet, close the door and leave the room.

☙❧

This trip is different from Jungle Doors, which reveals concrete stumbling blocks to weight loss, and Teddy Bear (the next trip), which reveals old irrational ideas about food. Instead, Emotional Closet reveals your feelings about food. Since feelings are much more difficult to define and sort out, the meaning of the things you see in your Emotional Closet may not be as instantly clear as they often are in other meta-images. Recognizing their importance may take some contemplation.

Thus, after doing this meta-image, we suggest you find a comfortable place and think about the experience. What kinds of things did you find in the closet? Are they directly related to food? Are these things just stored in the closet, or are they hidden? Could you be comfortable bringing them into the light of day? Were there particular foods in the closet? Were there people? Did you find the closet's contents helpful or detrimental to your weight-control efforts? Do the things that were in the closet relate to you as you are in the "here-and-now" at your age and stage of life, or do they relate to things that happened long ago from the "there-and-then"?

As you begin to deal with these questions, you can begin to work through some of the things in your emotional closet and discard those that are no longer useful to you or that get in your way. You can begin to make room for new feelings that can help you achieve permanent weight loss.

TEDDY BEAR

Purpose: To help you discard outmoded eating ideas and habits that you learned as a child, which are still contributing to your overweight.

❧

Picture yourself in a playroom. Image yourself as you look now sitting on the floor. You are dressed in clothes much like the ones you wore as a young child. Experience the total scene. In the room with you are a number of old, worn-out toys, each of them an eating idea, attitude, or habit that is no longer appropriate. In the corner you see a worn-out teddy bear. Go over to it and pick it up. You recognize it as one of these "toys." Notice what old idea or act it represents. The teddy bear may open its mouth and tell you, or it may be written on the toy somewhere. Ask yourself, "Am I ready to give this one up? If not now, when?" Go through the toys in this way until you are ready to discard one of them. When you find such a toy, throw it down. Then leave the playroom and close the door.

❧

Parents often unwittingly instill eating patterns that are detrimental in later life, for example by urging children to eat fast and eat everything they have been given, as if not eating will deprive starving people in foreign countries. Even though you know they are illogical, you still follow these internalized parental instructions. After you have done this meta-image, it would be helpful to write down which "teddy bear" you think it most important to erase, and how you can go about it. It is difficult and unnecessary to give them all up, or to give them all up at once. Start by being willing to give up just one of them; it will make a big difference. You can do the trip several times to become aware of other outmoded "teddy bears."

19

DEALING WITH SPECIFIC FOODS

CHAT WITH A FAMOUS PERSON

Purpose: To help you "mentally practice" ways of eating that will reduce your food consumption. In this trip you interrupt and delay your eating while you are involved in a fascinating conversation.

❧

Picture yourself at the dinner table. Where do you usually sit? What does the dining area look like, sound like? Food is on the table and you are beginning your main course. Pick up your fork, put a small amount of food into your mouth, chew and swallow it. Experience the sensation of your teeth moving against the food, the taste of the food in your mouth, the sensation of swallowing and having the food go down your throat and into your stomach. You are eating foods you enjoy. Continue until you have consumed about three-quarters of the food.

At this point, some famous and interesting person comes into the dining area and sits down in a chair opposite you. This person may be a living celebrity, someone from the past, or a character in a book or play. You and the famous person exchange greetings. You have many questions you want to ask, and the individual is genuinely interested in discussing them with you. Enjoy the give and take of the conversation. Note what the person looks like and sounds like, in addition to what he or she is saying. Fully experience the interesting conversation between yourself and this famous person. When you are ready, bid this person goodbye. You are now alone again with the remainder of your dinner. Complete your dinner if you feel like it.

❧

If you can actually stop, or at least interrupt, eating, it has been shown that the momentum driving you to overeat will diminish. Also, if you eat slowly and actually taste and savor your food you get much more out of it, which tends to deter overeating. After doing this meta-image, test it out by copying it in real life. When you next eat dinner, stop three-fourths of the way through the meal; pause for at least two to five minutes, and during that time recreate the conversation in your head, if you wish. Then continue eating until you feel satisfied. You are likely to eat less and enjoy it more.

SLOW MOTION

Purpose: To help you learn to slow down your eating, and to eat less in a restaurant, which for some people is a real problem. Our clients often say they lose weight eating at home or during the week, only to counteract it by overeating in restaurants, usually on the weekend. The net result is no weight loss and feelings of frustration and futility.

❧❧

Picture yourself entering your favorite restaurant. Image what the room looks like, what you are wearing, and whom you are with. Experience fully the sights, sounds, and smells in the restaurant. Picture yourself being shown to a table. Sit down at the table.

The waiter approaches your table and offers you a menu. You order something you enjoy and can "handle" calorie-wise. You feel good doing so. Feel the warm glow as you realize that you are in control and on top of the situation. Enjoy the conversation of the people you are with. Experience having an interesting conversation, sipping your water, and feeling completely relaxed.

The waiter now returns with your food. You notice something rather peculiar. At your table, time has slowed down. You are astonished to note that everything, except the conversation, is occurring in slow motion. It seems to take the waiter forever to place the plate in front of you. You see his hands perform a slow-motion ballet as the plate is put in front of you. You see his hands remain motionless. Slowly, slowly, you pick up your fork or spoon. Your motions seem graceful as you take some food and guide it into your mouth. Experience a great calmness as you eat in slow motion. Marvel at the feeling. You enjoy the relaxed pace. Look at the other diners around your table. They seem to be engaged in a race to finish; sparks are flying from their forks. The waiters are scurrying around. You return to your own oasis of calm and finish your meal in relaxed enjoyment.

If you go through this meta-image as a "rehearsal" before going out to eat, and then recreate the scene in the restaurant, you will find it has astonishing results. Our clients report they drastically slow down their eating with only a little mental practice. Their eating at restaurants, and in general, becomes calmer and more pleasant, no matter how crowded or hectic the eating place may be. Many people also report that after slow-motion practice, they drink less because they are more calm. Also, by slowing down you find that you need less food to feel satisfied, and often leave food on your plate. (If you have trouble with food sitting in front of you, unobtrusively salt it excessively or pour a little water on it to make it inedible.)

THE RABBIT

Purpose: This is a negative meta-image, designed to help you control compulsive eating of a specific food or in a certain eating situation. You'll want to use it less often than positive images, but if properly used, it will deter you from eating that you feel is harmful and that you can't at the moment seem to control any other way.

Picture yourself sitting somewhere by yourself. You are eating. You are overdosing on a particular food you love or just eating too much in general. You have already eaten enough to be full, and you know you've had enough, but you just keep on. You tell yourself you don't care, you'll diet tomorrow, anything—as you continue to eat. Suddenly you notice that a large white rabbit has hopped into the room. You are rather startled, but before you can move, the rabbit has settled itself right on top of the food. Watch the rabbit begin to nibble at the food you were eating just a minute ago. It eats rapidly, its mouth and nose moving up and down rapidly and rhythmically. You notice that the rabbit has a peculiar barnyard odor. You try to remove the animal, but it refuses to budge, and keeps on eating more and more. All of a sudden, the rabbit opens its mouth and throws up all over everything—all over the food, all over the table, all over you. You are horrified. You begin to feel nauseated; you get up from where you are and proceed to throw up.

Now say "Stop." Stop the scene and replace it with a pleasant, positive scene. You may want to use one of the positive mind trips in this book. You feel your stomach relaxing, your whole body loosening up, and the desire to continue to overeat completely gone.

You can make up variations on this scene using any number of animals. The point is to develop the meta-image vividly so you fully experience the greedy animal and its disgusting behavior. You can decide whether you want to image yourself throwing up. Many of our clients report that just the animal's vomiting is sufficient to stop them from continuing to eat compulsively.

IMMERSION

Purpose: If you have a particular food you can't handle, this meta-image will help you develop negative feelings toward it. The theory is that when we "overdo" something drastically, it tends to lose its attraction. Thus, in this trip, which is in two parts, you totally experience one of your problem foods, first by immersing yourself in it, and then eating so much you symbolically explode.

☙❧

Picture yourself inside a room. You see a very large amount of one of your favorite foods. Fill up a table with it. Now fill up the room. Remove your shoes and wade into the food. Walk through it and on it. Feel it on the bottoms of your feet and squishing through your toes. Now get down on all fours and crawl around in the food. See it and feel it oozing through your hands and under your knees. Rub it through your hair and over your face. Roll in the food. Grab a large handful and jam it into your mouth. It's dripping down your chin, sticking to the roof of your mouth, to your teeth. Take a second handful and continue shoving it into your mouth.

Now say "Stop" and relax. Open your eyes.

Close your eyes again. Bring into your mind some favorite place. Experience it. Now leave your favorite place and walk down a road. You come to a door. Notice what kind of door it is—of wood, metal, or what? Open the door. It opens easily. Behind the door is a table, piled high with your favorite food. There are mounds and mounds of the food, and the smell of it is filling the room.

Go to the table, lift up some of the food in your hand, and start to eat it. Continue to eat compulsively. You are getting full, but you realize you must eat until all of the food is gone. You can feel the skin around your mouth and jaws becoming stretched and painful. Your jaw aches and your stomach stretches from the strain. Now you can't see your feet, but you keep eating. You get larger and larger. The sides of your body are almost touching the walls of the room. You are blown up, but the food is only three-fourths gone. And you must eat it all. You can see your arm reaching for the food as your body gets larger and larger. You can no longer experience your neck; it is lost in folds of fat. Your abdomen has no shape. And your whole body hurts from the strain of accommodating the food. Your body now touches the ceiling as well.

The table is nearly empty, and you are reaching for the last bit of food. Your body now bursts, and parts of you are flying all over the room. Your hands fly across and hit the wall and bounce to the floor. Your head hits the light fixture on the ceiling. Completely image all of your parts exploding.

Quickly now, pull yourself together. Take all of your body parts and put them back together. Stick on your legs, arms, and head. Leave the room and walk rapidly down the road. You find yourself back in the body you started in, and you are relieved—but you know you must lose weight. With this realization, you feel calmer and more in control. You touch yourself to make sure you are really back in one piece. You are happy to note that your jaws no longer ache, and you can see your feet below you. Go to a place where you are calm and begin to feel totally, beautifully relaxed—at peace with the world and yourself.

In the future when you are faced with this food, flash into your mind the feeling you had when you overindulged—the nausea, the pain in your jaw, the tautness of your skin as you blew up. Then, if you reject the food in real life, experience the calm, restfulness, and well-being you felt at the end of the mind trip. You will find with practice you can bring forth the negative image rapidly to deter you from eating, and just as rapidly replace it with the positive one to make yourself feel good for eating appropriately.

This trip is very potent, so you should use it with care, only with foods that are really troublesome. One of our clients, for example, was a compulsive mashed potato eater; after this trip, she completely lost her taste for them. Another one of our clients used this trip to help him stop drinking calorie-laden liquor. During the trip, he hated the feeling of dizziness and the loss of all sensation as he continued to drink all the liquor in the room. For several months he could not bear to take a drink. Now, he can take a drink or two, but he uses this image to avoid drinking more than is good for him.

WORMS

Purpose: To specifically turn you off a certain food by making it seem noxious, unpleasant, or disgusting.

This is an "aversive" mind trip, which should be used sparingly. But there are times when you may want to make a food you are faced with seem undesirable or inedible.

❧❧

Picture yourself in a situation where you are faced with a food that often seems irresistible to you. Notice how great the food looks. Smell it. Begin to imagine how delicious it tastes. You can almost feel yourself eating it. Now, pick up some of the food, and put it in your mouth.

As you look down at what is left, you discover there are green oozy worms crawling out of the food. Watch them wiggle and squirm all over the food. It dawns on you that if there are worms crawling out of the food, there are green worms crawling around in your mouth, on the food you are eating. You begin to feel the worms crawling in your mouth, alive and moving. They are between your lips and coming out of your mouth. You can even smell them. They smell like spoiled meat.

They slither down your chin, and down the front of you. You are horrified and panicked as you see them wiggle down your clothes, leaving a foul mess. You begin to get very sick to your stomach. You throw it all up—the food, the worms, everything.

Now say "Stop." Eliminate the scene. Go to your "favorite place" until you feel relaxed and comfortable.

❧❧

The next time you want to avoid this food, call to mind this scene. Look at the food and image worms in it; recall how sick they made you feel. Some people after doing this mind trip, however, don't even have to avoid the food consciously. Whenever they see it they either feel no appetite at all or a slight nausea upon remembering, or associating, the worm images.

FOOD FIGHT

Purpose: When we feel pursued or overwhelmed by something, a constructive way to deal with it sometimes is to turn the tables and become the pursuer. In this meta-image, you turn and face your food "adversary" and vanquish it. This trip can also help you blow off emotional steam.

❧

Clearly bring into your mind a food you love to eat but have trouble coping with. What is its color, texture, smell? How do you think it will taste? Image a large amount of this food in front of you. Notice that the food starts to grow before your eyes. It gets larger and larger, until you are overshadowed by it.

You begin to get nervous as the food swells and becomes somewhat intimidating. It suddenly begins to move. You start to back away. The food moves forward at a rapid pace. You begin to run and it chases after you. You feel your heart pounding, your blood racing, and your throat dry as you try to escape your pursuer. You become increasingly afraid that the food will catch and overwhelm you. The more frightened and desperate you get, the more relentlessly the food pursues you. Experience the food pursuing you like some science-fiction monster.

Now stop in your tracks. Take a deep breath,

hold it for a few seconds, and slowly let it out. As you do, you feel yourself becoming strong, calm, and effective. Turn and face your "monster." It seems to have shrunk somewhat in size. You are seized with an urge to demolish it. Picture yourself kicking and punching the food. Feel your foot come in contact with the blob of food. Experience the power in your arm as you land a lightning-quick blow. Pick up a stick now. Hit the food again, and again and again . . . beat it up until it is shrunken in size, until you are feeling better and no longer upset. Now step back and look at the food lying there. It is in a heap, formless and totally unappetizing. You wonder now how it could ever have appealed to you or seemed to have such power over you.

You may find, as others have, that this trip is quite liberating and produces a great sense of satisfaction. It allows you to express hostile feelings toward a food harmlessly with victorious results. People who have done this trip in the middle of compulsive desires to continue eating have reported that it dramatically stopped the binge in a matter of moments. One woman who lost 30 pounds in our program—and kept it off—used the image to fight it out with a batch of cupcakes in her kitchen. She was so disgusted with them, and herself for wanting to eat them, that she mashed them "to death" on the kitchen floor.

Some people say they have trouble getting the food to lie still, that it begins moving or breathing, as if coming back to life. Another woman reported that while beating on a "monster" caramel her stick got stuck, so her blows were less effective. This is not important. Remember, you control the images—they are happening as you direct them to happen. You need not expect the food to be totally "dead." You may not be ready for that yet; or it may not be necessary for you in the context of your eating problem. You are doing what you are willing to do at the moment. For some, just turning on the food and "facing it down" can be a tremendous victory that brings significant results in actually handling the food. Sometimes you may have to repeat the image a few times before you are *completely* in control.

METAMORPHOSIS

Purpose: It can often help if you are obsessed by a certain food to *become* your obsession. This trip allows you to image changing yourself into a food. Thus, you experience it from a different perspective and may come to think about it differently. The meta-image also allows you to continue to think about food, but in a new, diverting fashion, which may deter you from eating.

Picture a particular food that you love. A food that you might compulsively eat. Now begin to experience becoming that food. Feel your body as it changes into the obsessed food. Experience the texture, density, color, shape, temperature. Notice where you are located: on a plate, on a shelf, in a refrigerator, in a bakery, looking out from a super-market aisle, or where? Are you packaged in any way? Notice all the things in your environment.

Fully experience how it feels to be that food. Continue the imagery until you feel like concluding it.

❧❦

This is an excellent meta-image to do when you feel you lack control handling a certain food. When tempted to eat the food, you can do the Metamorphosis instead; this may defuse the food's attraction much the same way actually contemplating a food will do. You'll recall that when meticulously scrutinized, a food often loses its appeal.

One man used this trip to help control his overeating of ice cream. He experienced himself as the food in a freezer—dark, unhappy, and trapped. He felt himself being irritated by the abrasive almonds in him and his sweet, sugary taste. Another woman saw herself as a doughnut being carried around all day in the pocket of a little girl. Whenever the woman thought of eating such a doughnut, she usually didn't, because she knew how disappointed the little girl would be to reach in her pocket and find the doughnut missing. Crazy? Perhaps a little. But it only illustrates the amazing potential of the human mind to monitor actions—and it works!

BALLOONS

Purpose: To help you eat normally, without overindulging, when you go to a party or other place where quantities of attractive food are available for the taking. The first part of the trip, in which you focus on the food at the expense of everything else, is negative. It is followed by a positive trip, where you experience the good feeling of being in control of your eating, which will carry over to real-life situations. The positive trip also helps you "rehearse" or "mentally practice" how you want to eat at a party, thus helping break old habits and reinforcing a new, more appropriate style of eating.

Picture yourself in an area where a party is going on. Notice what you are wearing, what you look like in it, who is with you, who the other people there are, what they are saying and doing. Now image a tableful of food and move toward it. Picture all of the foods you are likely to find at a party. Image how they look and smell. Begin to eat. Take a large amount of food. Pile it on your plate. Now, with rapid motions, your head bent over the plate, eat everything on it. Now return to the food and refill your plate. As you do so, edge other people away from the food, practically snatching it out of their hands. People begin to have peculiar looks on their faces, but you pay no attention, and devote yourself to piling the food on your plate. Rapidly put the food in your mouth. Feel yourself belting down the food, mindless of its taste.

Someone comes up to you and begins a conversation. It is someone interesting you want to talk with. But to your horror, you find you cannot stop the hand-to-mouth movement. You try, but the harder you try, the faster you are eating. You talk while eating. The food particles fall out of your mouth. The person retreats. You are mortified. Now you are getting very full and people are beginning to stare at you. You continue to eat compulsively. You begin to blow up. You get larger and rounder like a balloon. By this time, everyone at the party is staring at you openly. You can only guess what they are thinking about you. You blow up bigger and bigger, and find yourself floating, rising like some giant balloon—but you are still eating. You drift closer and closer to a large open window and begin to float out of it and upward. You are terrified by now. You wish fervently you could do something to stop eating. You feel like a balloon, floating out and about to burst. Now say "Stop." Stop the image. Begin again.

Picture yourself just outside the door, ready to enter the party. Notice what you are wearing. Are you with anyone? Your host or hostess meets you at the door and expresses pleasure at your being able to come. You smile, express your thanks, and enter the room. What does it look like? Who is there? What are they saying and doing?

You see the food and move toward it. Take an average amount of the foods you really enjoy. Then move away from the location of the food. Place a bite in your mouth, and chew it slowly, really "tasting" the food. Notice its texture, its flavor. Savor it. Someone interesting moves toward you and you begin a conversation. You slowly eat the food, talk, move about the room, and focus on the people rather than the food. You feel yourself in control of the situation. You begin to feel yourself getting slimmer and more attractive with each step you take. Both men and women respond to you positively. You feel good, and enjoy the party. Experience the positive self-feelings in this party scene. When you have had enough, open your eyes.

Note how different you felt in the two scenes. When you feel positive about yourself and other people, food becomes secondary. Whenever you know you will be confronted with a difficult party situation, where you may overeat, mentally practice the second party scene before you go; you'll find you *will* begin to conform to the image of yourself in the mind trip.

INNER EATING

Purpose: This is a most remarkable trip in which you fool your mind into believing you are eating a food when you are consuming only the image of the food. You thus eat the food purely in your mind to the point of feeling full and satisfied so that the desire for the food vanishes. It is the ultimate in calorie-free eating. The reason it works, of course, is that nearly always your hunger is "mind hunger" to begin with and not true physical "body hunger." It won't work if you are *physically* hungry.

❧

Picture a food you have a craving for. Clearly focus on it. Now pick it up, put it in your mouth, and go through all the motions and feelings of eating it. Roll it around on your tongue and experience the taste. Enjoy chewing, sucking, or licking it. Feel it go slowly down your throat. Continue to eat it in your usual fashion until you have had enough or it is gone. Experience feeling full and satisfied.

❧

If done completely and vividly, so that you actually *experience* eating the food, this trip can be fantastic—and it is, for some people. But there is a caution: If you fail to experience it fully, you may find that it acts as a mental "rehearsal" or a sensitizer heightening your desire for the food. For some it is possible to do this trip and end up "longing" for the food. If that happens it would be wise to discontinue using this trip. There is a difference between *saying* you hear a dog barking and actually *hearing* a dog barking in imagery, as we pointed out earlier in the book.

Even if you do this trip effectively, it does not mean you will never eat the food in reality—but probably you will eat it less often. One woman who likes a hot fudge sundae made by a certain ice-cream parlor actually eats one about every three weeks. This is how she says she deals with her cravings for the sundae in the interim:

"I was sitting in the den thinking about having a hot fudge sundae, which I adore, but calorie-wise is a disaster. Instead, I see myself at my favorite ice-cream parlor sitting in a booth. I am handed a menu and tell the waitress I don't need it. I am ordering a hot fudge sundae with vanilla fudge ice cream and peanuts scattered on top. I look around and drink some cold water. It feels good going down and helps me handle my impatience. The sundae finally is here. I can see the steam rise slightly on the thick brown fudge, as it slides slowly down the sides, mixing with and making little puddles in the ice-cream dish. I put my hand around the dish. It feels cold and nice. I like that feeling. I pick up the spoon and run it around the rim of the dish, picking up some of the spilled fudge. I put it in my mouth. The sweet taste explodes inside my mouth. I am eating it slowly now. The peanuts crunch with the cold ice cream. It is impossible to describe. I just eat it slowly, savoring every spoonful right to the bottom of the dish. What's so incredible is that I've thought about going for a sundae every day now for three weeks, but after eating it this way, I feel like I've really eaten it, and the craving goes away."

20

FINDING SOLUTIONS

PRISONER

Purpose: Somewhere inside you may already know what would help you lose weight, but are unaware of your inner knowledge. This meta-image will help unlock those inner solutions that you already possess.

❧

Picture yourself in a jail cell. It is a prison you have made for yourself by your eating habits: rapid eating, bingeing, eating on the run, eating without tasting. It represents all the previous failures and feelings of frustration and hopelessness that engulf you when you think about your weight. You sit in your cell thinking about these things. Slowly you begin to realize that you must zero in on the solution, not the problem. You begin to think about a key. Imagé a large key to open the padlock of the jail cell you have created. Something is engraved on the key that is a solution to your weight problems. Allow whatever comes to mind to appear on the key. Notice what it is. Now take the key and insert it in the lock of your cell and open the door. See yourself coming out of the cell weighing less than when you went in.

❧❧

Since there are many different solutions to your eating problem, image as many keys as you need to, unlocking as many cells as are necessary. You'll find that the next time you're faced with an eating problem, if you image the large key, you may immediately "see" the solution.

THE SCALE

Purpose: This is one of the most simple, popular, and *potent* trips. It gives you a weight-loss goal that you can constantly and easily flash into your mind. When you do that, it is amazing how effective it is in deterring you from overeating.

❧❧

Picture a scale, the kind of step-on scale you would find in a doctor's office, with weights and a balance bar. Picture yourself nude, getting on the scale and moving the weights until the bar is balanced and you can read your current weight. How do you feel about it? What are you saying to yourself now? Make the scene as vivid as you can. Say "Stop." Go back to the beginning, seeing yourself once again in the nude and stepping on to the scale. This time, however, when you move the weights to balance the bar, you will be able to read your desired weight on the scale. This will be a good and normal weight, not too thin, not too fat, realistically right for you. Experience how it feels to read this new weight. Pay particular attention to your inner dialogue. Now see yourself leaving the scale and getting dressed.

※※

Before or as you start to eat you can bring the second part of the meta-image to mind—seeing yourself on the scale with the weight registering what you wish. You can also flash it into your mind with every few bites. When you're actually eating, your thoughts may shift back and forth between the scale image of your old weight and future weight, but that's all right as long as you always remember to finish with the second positive image of the thinner you.

The image is powerful because it helps you focus vividly on the consequences of eating *before* you overdo it. Too often—in fact, *most* often—overeaters impulsively eat and then think of the consequences only later. It also works because it gives you a good positive feeling about yourself. Every time you flash it, you recreate how great you felt when you actually saw the scale balance at your hoped-for weight. That mild but positive psychic reward can be a potent motivator on its own.

NEWSREEL

Purpose: To let you examine some of your present eating actions and then devise an opposite way of eating. Before the advent of television, the movie houses used to show a five-minute documentary film of news, called a newsreel. In this trip, you watch such a newsreel about yourself. First, you may want to think about specific instances in which you overeat—at home alone at night, at parties, while watching television, when upset, etc.

❧

Picture yourself entering a movie theater. The screen is blank, the lights are on. What does this theater look like? What colors, what smells, what sounds? See yourself move down the aisle toward a seat and sit down. The lights dim, the music starts, and the show begins with the newsreel, the news of the day. This news is about you and your eating problem. The news reports how you usually behave, where you are, what you're doing, what you're thinking. Watch your news story until it reaches your usual ending. Zero in on what you feel. Now say "Stop."

The screen darkens and you can hear the sound of the film rewinding. Now the news starts again from the beginning. The scene is the same, but what you are doing, what's happening, and the outcome is the *opposite* of what you saw before. Allow this newsreel to run until it ends. When it is over, ask yourself what has changed. What is the new outcome and how do you feel about it? Run as many different newsreels as you like until you feel you have done all the possible opposites of the original troublesome scene. Then choose the scene that you feel is most likely to be successful. Watch this new scenario a number of times until you become familiar with it.

※

This newsreel lets you "rehearse" new ways of eating. Thus, if you practice it enough so you really know it, you will find that when faced with an eating problem, you can rerun the desired eating part of the newsreel in your head—while *at the same time* acting it out in real life. You will find it works. Many people in our program have been astounded to find that the "rehearsal" in their heads does translate to action in the real world.

STAIRCASE

Purpose: To help you "see" a particular goal in losing weight and to help you devise specific steps to reaching it.

※

Picture a staircase. Notice where it is located, what it is made of, what kind it is, how many steps there are.

Now see a weight-loss-related goal at the top of the stairs. Put one foot on the first step of the stairs. Test it for firmness. Go up another step. Slowly, one step at a time, move up the stairs. As you go up each step, repeat to yourself some phrase that can help you lose weight. When you reach the top, take joy in your accomplishment. Feel yourself standing at the top of the stairs exhilarated. Experience your success fully.

It will be interesting to notice what kind of staircase you created. The stairway is more effective if it is realistic, one you can actually climb. Sometimes, people who can't conceive of reaching their goals create long, interminable staircases with only a hazy goal seen from a long distance.

As others have noted, your style may be revealed by the way you go about climbing the stairs. One adolescent girl in our program imaged a rickety staircase and was never able to make it to the top. As she was about to take the last step, her staircase dissolved. She approached dealing with her weight in much the same way. She lost a pound or two, but had difficulty focusing on a long-range goal. In fourteen weeks, her weight fluctuated between losing 12 pounds and gaining 10.

A very successful teenager was at first frightened when she saw her overweight mother on the top step. She was able to replace that image with one of herself in a new thinner body. She continued to lose about a pound a week until now she is of normal weight.

FIRST-AID KIT

Purpose: When you are faced with a situation in which you might overeat, one way to overcome the desire is to reach into your mind and come up with pleasing mental images that can distract you, giving you something else to focus on instead of eating. But the images must be instantly available so you can flash them into your mind. This meta-image helps you create a "first-aid" emergency kit full of interesting diversions which you can turn to in difficult eating situations.

❧

Picture yourself in a room in your house other than the kitchen, a room where you are very comfortable and where you like to be. Experience where you are in the room. Is it warm or cool? What is the furniture like? How is the room decorated? Can you hear any sounds? Make the experience as vivid as you possibly can. Now you are going to prepare an emergency box full of things you like to help you during difficult eating situations.

Image finding a box of some sort, at least as large as a shoe box, or larger if you wish. Picture putting in all kinds of things that give you pleasure. Picture yourself putting in a loved object, an object that makes you happy when you look at it, touch it, or use it. Put in a book you might enjoy reading. Put in the telephone number of someone special—someone who makes you feel good when you call. Put in a picture of a place that you have been where you were really happy and comfortable. Put in something nice that someone once said about you that you liked hearing. Put in something nice that you can say about yourself. Put in an accomplishment, something that you have achieved that makes you feel really good about yourself. Put in toys, games, anything you like. Now put the box containing all of these things away in a special place so you can quickly get it when you need it.

❧❧

There is virtually no end to the fascinating things you might put in such an emergency box. One woman keeps an imaginary yo-yo in her kit which she mentally "plays" with when she needs to escape situations in which everyone around her is eating. Nor is food out of place in the kit. One man, for instance, carries in his kit his ideal image of a chocolate-chip cookie, which he looks at occasionally.

Some people in our program have set up real first-aid kits to divert them when food "calls." But, interestingly, many could not think of what to put in their boxes until they took the mind trip to discover, indeed, what they find pleasurable. The trip freed them to be creative.

MENTAL GARDEN

Purpose: We all harbor some ideas, notions, and myths which are no longer helpful or useful to us. In fact, many were never accurate to begin with. This is particularly true about myths related to weight control. This image is designed to help you view some of these myths as if they were weeds in a garden, and to pull them out. Symbolically removing the mistaken beliefs from your "mental garden" may also uproot them at another level of your consciousness, weakening or destroying the influence on your actions. And your chances of succeeding at permanently losing weight will increase.

The mistaken beliefs that cause weight-loss failure to be uprooted in this meta-image are the effectiveness of crash dieting, denial, will power, and the notion that thin people are always happy.

It's a sunny, beautiful May day and you are in a lovely garden. See the clusters of flowers, hear the birds, smell the grass, feel the warmth of the sun. Make the garden image as vivid as you can. Concentrate on the plants and flowers in the garden. What are the different varieties? What kind of flowers, what kind of shrubbery do you see? Put whatever you wish into your garden.

Now walk to the end of the garden, and to your dismay, you find a corner that is badly in need of weeding. See yourself starting to pull out these weeds. The first clump of weeds has been in the garden a long time, so it will take a lot of effort to pull it out, to uproot the idea it represents—"Crash Dieting Will Get Me There." See yourself grappling with it and pulling it out root and all. Move on to the next growth of weeds in your garden. This weed says, "Thin People Are Happy." Root out this mistaken belief as you pull out the weeds. You come to the third patch of weeds. They are very, very old and they have been there a long time, and you really have to work to get rid of the weeds known as "Will Power Is Necessary." You pull and tug until these weeds are out. Be careful with the next bunch of weeds. If you let them grow in your garden they can poison you. They are called "Denial Is Required to Lose Weight." As you rip out the denial weed, feel the perspiration trickling down your body. Your arms are taut and you are straining every muscle. Tug at the weed and feel it finally give way. Now gather up all the weeds you have pulled and throw them away.

❧❧

To refresh your memory, here in capsule form are the reasons that the four myths are destructive of efforts to lose weight.

1. "Crash Dieting Will Get Me There." When this belief persists, you go on a crash diet, lose weight, and then regain it. In the end, you have had one more negative, failure-producing experience.

2. "Thin People Are Happy." If you believe the myth that thin people are happy, what you are really saying is, "If I get thin, I will miraculously be happy like all of those other thin people." That's not really true. Normal-weight people are just normal weight. They have some of the same problems, feelings, attitudes that overweight people do, but they handle their problems in other ways rather than turning to food.

3. "Will Power Is Necessary." We have found that will power is a negative concept, particularly since people tend to believe that the lack of it is a character flaw. It's not. Will power can be counterproductive in permanently losing weight.

4. "Denial Is Required to Lose Weight." We have found that when people deny themselves certain foods they have a great deal of difficulty. You can learn to eat everything. There is no forbidden food. There are no inappropriate foods, only inappropriate *amounts* of food. Denial usually builds up a craving for forbidden foods, and most people on a denial regimen last only so long before they succumb.

FORTUNE COOKIE

Purpose: There are certain phrases or ideas that, if kept in mind, can be enormously helpful in losing weight. In Mental Garden you uproot some erroneous beliefs that prevent you from losing weight. In Fortune Cookie you can implant new rational concepts that will help you lose weight. If you use this meta-image enough, the statements will begin to automatically pop into your mind, deterring you from overeating.

Picture yourself at a very nice Chinese restaurant. It may or may not be one you have been to before. Look at the surroundings, smell the food, listen to the sounds typical of a fine Chinese restaurant. You and your companion are sitting in a booth or at a table. Image eating your dinner, enjoying the food, eating it slowly. You can see yourself eating small amounts, putting your fork down between bites. You are with someone you want to be with, you are enjoying the conversation, savoring the food, sipping the tea, feeling comfortable and happy.

After the main course the waiter brings you three fortune cookies. Now you are curious; you wonder what message is in each of them. Start to open the first one. The brittle cookie begins to crumble with a cracking sound. You pull out a little blue slip of paper on which is a small typed sentence: "I am fatter than I am hungry." You smile a little, shake your head, and recognize that this is true; that very often you know you are eating when you are not hungry.

Now reach for the second fortune cookie. Open it and extract the little piece of paper. It says, "I can eat two tablespoons of anything." You think about it for a second and you agree that you won't gain weight from any food if you eat it in moderation.

Now you break open the third fortune cookie. Its message is, "I can always eat it tomorrow." And you know that in most instances that's true. The same food will be available to you again. This is not your last chance to have it.

Now take these three pieces of paper and put them in your purse or in your wallet.

You now have these statements in your mental purse or wallet and can take them out and look at them whenever you need or want to. You might also want to image exactly where they are in your purse or wallet, and think about them whenever you actually open your purse or wallet. Thus they will act as constant reminders of how to lose weight successfully.

X-RAY

Purpose: This trip gives you something to think about when you are eating by focusing your attention on what happens to food in the body. If you mentally follow every bite of food's progress through your body, you can considerably slow down your eating. The trip also increases your awareness of the purpose of food and of the fact that eating does not end in the mouth.

Picture a food that you like. Pick it up, and put some of it in your mouth. Feel your teeth chewing it. As it mixes with saliva, it changes slowly to liquid form. See it slide down your throat. Now see it pass by your organs on its way to your stomach. Notice any contractions and secretions. The food moves out to give your body sustenance, and into yards and yards of tangled intestines. Now see it in a form to be evacuated. Follow the complete trip of the food through your body.

This is a trip you can practice and then flash into your mind when you are actually eating.

Since it is an awareness trip, it doesn't matter whether your imaging is physiologically correct. It can be most fanciful and still make its point. Your visualization of how your body functions will depend on your knowledge, feelings, and beliefs. For some, this is a slightly aversive trip when they think of the food they are eating being turned into excrement. Others have actually seen the food they are eating turn into fat globules and race around the body looking for a place to attach themselves. Thus they witness the fat accumulation at the instant they are creating it, and it sometimes curtails their eating.

However, many find the trip pleasant and use it only to slow down their rate of eating.

21

DEVELOPING A BETTER BODY IMAGE

SELF-PORTRAITS

Purpose: To implant a picture of a slimmer you in your mind, a picture toward which you will then move. It also helps you to see realistically how you look now as well as to project the image of how you want to look and how you can look.

❧❧

    Picture yourself in an art gallery. It is quiet, restful, and you are walking along, enjoying the paintings on the wall. As you approach one of the paintings, you see that it is a full-length, life-sized portrait of you and the way you look now. Examine the portrait. Carefully, go over the face, the head, the arms, the trunk. Notice the texture of the skin. Are you nude, or wearing clothes? What kind of clothing? How does it fit? How do you look in it? Notice that the artist has made a realistic appraisal of your whole body. Are you comfortable and pleased with it? Would other people find it pleasant or unpleasant to look at? After you have examined your portrait from head to toe, move on.

As you walk, you notice other paintings along the gallery wall. Now, you come upon another portrait of yourself painted by the same artist. It is a portrait of you as you would like to look—and could expect to look if you ate properly. It is a portrait of you in the future. Examine it carefully, as you did the other one. Notice the differences. And realize that this is the way you can realistically expect to look in the future if you eat appropriately. Now image yourself moving into this picture, becoming one with the second portrait. Experience how good it feels to be the second "slimmer" you.

❧

Some people with weight problems have a distorted perception of what their bodies really look like; they may avoid mirrors and photographs. One of our clients was totally disbelieving when a friend pointed out another woman similar in body build. She exclaimed: "But she's dumpy and fat. I don't look like that." But she did. Doing this mind trip helped her bring her true body image into focus, and see that it was not as she desired to look. Subsequently, she lost 22 pounds.

It is important, however, not to dwell on the first portrait, but on the second, slimmer, healthier you.

You can flash this image regularly into your mind when you feel you may overeat. Just the mind picture of what you can and will look like if you don't overeat can act as a powerful reinforcer to proper eating, and give you control over your eating.

BEACH DOORS

Purpose: Sometimes it is difficult to like or accept your body, and this can block weight loss. This meta-image lets you discover things about your body that you can accept, thus helping you realize a more positive body image.

Picture yourself floating in the water somewhere, moving lazily and pleasantly toward shore. You reach the beach and start walking away from the shore toward a different land scene. Allow yourself to experience the climate, the sun, the breeze on your body, or whatever is present for you in the scene. As you walk, you are quite comfortable, quite curious; you look around and enjoy what you are seeing. You come upon a door, and you know that behind that door is an aspect of your body you like or can accept. Now open the door and experience whatever is there. Go through the door and continue walking. Farther along, you come to a second door. And you say, "Oh, here's another door, and behind that there's something else I like or accept about my body." Open the door and experience whatever you find behind the second door. Open as many doors as you can in this way.

People often feel: "I'm fat, therefore I'm worthless." It is important to remember you *have* a body; you are not your body. You are the sum total of many things, *including* your body. It is erroneous thinking to invest all of your self-worth in your body. There are probably aspects of your body that may never be as you now wish, no matter how much weight you lose. Thus, you will be more successful if you learn to accept the aspects of your body you cannot change.

There is always something you can find to like about your body. As one formerly fat woman says: "Even when I was fat, I loved my eyes." Recognizing one or a few things about your body that you like enhances your body image. As you grow more self-confident and lose weight, you will begin to accept and value your body more. You can do this Beach Doors meta-image regularly to check on what body-image progress you are making.

SKIN-ZIP

Purpose: Since many people have misconceptions about how it will feel to be of normal weight permanently, this trip helps you prepare for that day by letting you "try on" other bodies so you can see how you feel. The trip also helps you develop a more positive or realistic attitude toward your own body.

Picture yourself as a presence, a being, a body temporarily without a skin, but this is not unpleasant. As you move through space, you realize you are in an enclosed area, a large warehouse.

You can smell the mustiness associated with a warehouse. Experience being there, feeling it, sensing it, smelling it, invisibly walking across the floor. You come to an open space and see a long clothes rack filled with hangers and clothing. Curiously, you move closer and you can see that there are various "skin suits" on the hangers. There in front of you are the bodies, the outer coverings, of many different people. Each suit has a zipper that goes all the way around it. Look them over carefully. Some suits are the bodies of members of your family, others are of friends or acquaintances of yours. You may find television personalities, famous people, fictional characters, perhaps even cartoon characters. Give yourself plenty of time to inspect each of the skins. Handle each one on its hanger. Intrigued by the whole experience, you notice the physical characteristics of each "skin suit." The hangers scrape against the pole as you move each one aside. After going through them all, pick one out and put it on. Listen to the sound of the zipper as you enclose yourself in this other person's skin. Feel yourself begin to *be* the person whose body you have chosen. Experience his or her body movements. Is the body light and quick? Do you move rapidly in it? How does it feel to be in this new body? Are you happier or any sadder? Look smarter? Are you more in tune with the world? Are you friendlier, are you more loved? Experience the world from within this body for as long as you like. When you feel you have done so fully, take it off. Put it back on its hanger. Zip into your own skin and leave.

After you do this image, you will want to think about how realistic your expectations are. What would happen to you if you were in a body that seems more desirable to you than your own? One of our clients chose the body of Gina Lolabrigida, but upon analyzing her experiencing of the image, she decided that she would still prefer to live her own life and be herself. She also discovered that she would not like to be admired solely for her "looks." She moved on toward a better acceptance of herself as a person, and continued to lose weight.

However, if you like the way you felt in the body of your choice you might try to recreate that feeling in your own body. Try to act the way you think your borrowed body would act, if that pleases you. You can learn to model or imitate any trait you admire, and, of course, you can do this image any number of times, zipping yourself up into as many different skin suits as you wish.

22

HANDLING YOUR FEELINGS

COURTROOM

Purpose: This is an amazingly effective image that lets you give yourself a trial when you feel guilty about something. Through the imaginary trial you can purge yourself of guilt so you don't continue to carry it around as emotional baggage. The trial also helps put your so-called crime in proper perspective.

It's best for losing weight if you use this trip after a guilt-producing food-related situation, as when you overeat. But you can also use it to alleviate other types of guilty feelings that might induce you to overeat.

❧

First, picture a recent food-related episode about which you felt guilty or upset. Recreate the whole thing in your head. Stay with it until you have replayed it all. What was the situation? Who was there? What was said or done? How did you feel about it?

Now picture a courtroom. You are on trial for your unfortunate behavior. Using all of the senses—hearing, sight, sound, touch, and smell—put yourself in that courtroom. Picture the judge, the attorney who will defend you, the prosecuting attorney, the members of the jury. The trial begins. The prosecuting attorney states the case against you. Listen closely as he describes your "crime" to the judge and jury. Now your attorney defends you. He offers reasons and extenuating circumstances, if any, for your eating "crime." Everyone, including yourself, listens intently.

After all of the arguments have been presented, send the jury out to deliberate. When the jury returns, the foreman reads the verdict. If the verdict is "guilty," the judge passes sentence.

The trial ends.

❧

Afterward, reflect on your trial. Ask yourself if your "crime" was as great as you thought it was. Often people are much more harsh on themselves than any logic would dictate. Were the arguments presented by each lawyer realistic? Was there much exaggeration? If you are pronounced guilty, is the judge's sentence either too harsh or too lenient?

Some people have sentenced themselves to the most irrational severe sentences for minor eating infractions. For example, one woman in our program actually heard the judge say "death by hanging." This gave her a new insight into how demanding and critical she was of herself and her family. Subsequently, she began getting less upset about family behavior that was leading her to eat, and more tolerant of herself. The type of punishment you give yourself may reveal much about your temperament.

You may also want to notice who the judge, jury, and prosecutor turn out to be. Sometimes they are members of your family, friends, or famous figures. One man's defending attorney was King Henry VIII, who argued eloquently about the joys of food. The jury still found the defendant guilty.

Some people even manage to plead their cases further. One woman sentenced to "fifteen unhappy days" thought this unfair, and was surprised to see herself jump up and ask for "three unhappy days" and probation. The judge agreed, and since she had already been unhappy for three days, she emerged from the trial already having served her sentence. She felt a great sense of freedom and release.

If the sentence passed does seem realistic to you, then consider actually serving it. Many people find a reasonable self-punishment liberating. Many are also pleasantly surprised to find that the verdict is "not guilty."

Essentially, this trip helps you get your self-punishment and recriminations over with, finished, so you can *forget* about them. Then they don't interfere with your ongoing life and lead to additional overeating.

Truly, with this trip, you will see how remarkable your own mind is at solving problems and help-ing you resolve emotional conflicts.

TYPHOON

Purpose: To help you learn to ride out emotional "storms" without resorting to food as an escape hatch. It works best when you allow your imagina-tion to develop a raging, roaring South Seas storm such as you probably have seen in the movies.

※

Picture yourself somewhere on an island in the South Pacific. It is evening and you are standing on the beach, looking out at the ocean. Experience the total scene. Walk back toward a hut which is a little way back on the beach. Go through the front door. What does the room look like? What things are there? Spend some time imaging the total situation. Include all of your senses—sight, smell, sound, touch—to put you there.

Suddenly a wind comes up, seemingly out of nowhere. The sky begins to darken. You wonder if there will be a storm. You are worried. What if it should be a bad one, such as the typhoons you have heard people whispering about? The wind begins to howl and the trees start swaying dangerously. It be-gins to rain. As you listen, the rain begins to fall faster and harder. You think you should have headed for the mainland when it started. Now it is too late. You can feel yourself panicking. Your palms are sweaty, your throat dry. You can feel your heart pounding, and there is a knot in your stomach. You begin to panic. The winds rise higher, threatening to overtake everything. In a panic, you sit on the floor of the hut and wonder if you will survive. You begin to feel hungry and wonder if it is safe to get up and eat something.

Take a deep breath while sitting there on the floor of the hut. Don't bother to eat anything; that won't help deal with the anxiety. Instead slowly come to know that you will be all right. The storm will subside if you can only somehow live with the anxiety you feel. Tell yourself that you will allow yourself to feel this anxiety—that it doesn't have to be overwhelming. Say to yourself that the tension and anxiety will pass, that you can wait it out with the typhoon. Feel the anxiety now wash *over* you, not *through* you. You are in control of yourself. You can feel your body relax as you make the decision to spend the night listening to the wind and waiting for the dawn.

Often if you will *allow* yourself to feel tense and anxious, the feelings will diminish. It is possible to do this if you adopt the attitude that you can be anxious and survive it. Tension is often a reasonable feeling in many circumstances. Not to feel it would be unusual. But many people have noted that when they stop trying to fight their feelings and allow for them as just feelings (neither good nor bad), they are better able to cope. People find themselves free to come up with creative solutions to problems when they learn to "tolerate" levels of tension. At the very least, they often report a decrease in anxiety-produced eating.

Question to ask yourself: Were you able to ride out the storm without eating?

KARATE

Purpose: Often you may feel pent-up anger or aggression toward someone which you don't want to express fully. In this meta-image you can challenge your adversary to a fair, highly structured, supervised fight—and win, if you wish—without anyone getting hurt. Such an imaginary fight may diminish your anger and/or give you an interval to cool off until you can deal with the anger more directly.

If you are very upset, you may need to do a complete "body relaxation" before beginning the trip. Sometimes a few deep breaths, held and slowly released, will calm you down enough so you can get into the imagery.

Picture yourself in a karate studio. It is a large room with dressing rooms at one end and a mirror on the opposite wall. The walls are painted a soft, light color. There are mats strewn about the room. Sunlight is streaming through the windows, making patterns on the floor. Experience being in the room.

Your karate instructor greets you. He bows and introduces your opponent. You are surprised to see that this is the person you are upset with. You mumble a recognition, and then each of you goes into a dressing room to put on karate suits. You return wearing a white karate suit tied with a colored belt around your middle. Your opponent also comes out in a karate suit, and you bow to each other.

Now begins the karate combat.

Land a blow to the head, a chop to the stomach. Using your hands and feet, pummel the person until he or she gives up. Continue until the person is lying on the floor defeated, and you're satisfied. Your karate instructor commends you on your mastery. You thank the instructor, bowing, and state that the person upset you and you are glad you won. Allow the scene to fade, and open your eyes.

❧❧

This trip illustrates that the mind is a marvelous sanctuary where you can work out things free of actual consequences. What makes this image especially effective is that it is carefully constructed to give rules to the combat so as to make it acceptable. Some people in our program who use it regularly find it fantastic; but some others still say they "can't" do it because they feel guilty about expressing physical violence even in a mental game situation.

Certainly, there are times when direct expression of anger is appropriate and necessary. But many people are afraid of their anger because they let it build up to explosive proportions, so that in a confrontation it is apt to get out of hand, causing minor arguments to escalate into major battles. What the karate trip can do is take the edge off the anger or aggression, defusing it to an extent, making it easier to handle an actual confrontation. For example, one woman in our program used to become angry when her son came home at two in the morning. She used to deal with her anger by getting up and eating. However, when she saw her son the next morning she was still so angry she exploded, which led her to eat even more. Now, when she is angry at him, she does the karate trip, which curtails the eating. Having harmlessly vented her anger, she also finds she is much more in control and can conduct a reasonable discussion with him at the proper time.

PRESSURE COOKER

Purpose: To allow you to blow off steam when you need to, relieving feelings of frustration that could cause you to overeat.

❧❧

Picture yourself as a pressure cooker, a metal pot with a valve at the top that lets off steam in controlled amounts. Experience yourself as a big shiny metal pot. Feel the lid being clamped on. Now, you feel the heat being applied beneath you. Feel yourself getting warmer and warmer as the steam builds up inside you. Your pressure-cooker valve begins to jiggle; you can hear and feel it. Now you are feeling the steam slowly being channeled out through the top. It rises inside you and seeps out in small, steady, hissing streams. When all the steam is gone, and you have cooled down somewhat, someone comes and removes your lid. You feel free and comfortable.

❧❧

It's all right in this meta-image, too, if you let the whole lid blow off, or the cooker explode. For some people that is necessary to prevent them from blowing their lid in real life.

In psychology, there really is a "potboiler" theory of the expression of anger and aggression, called the "catharsis hypothesis." If you put a pot on the stove, and turn up the heat (anger, etc.), and at the same time hold down the lid (expression of these feelings), the steam pressure will build so there will be an eventual explosion. However, if you let the anger out a little at a time by lifting the lid occasionally, the likelihood of an explosion is lessened.

Unable to let off steam, some food-involved people cope with unexpressed feelings by overeating. It is an attempt to narcotize themselves with food. It doesn't work. It is far better to release the anger in acceptable ways as you go along.

LETTING GO

Purpose: Many people find they feel burdened and restrained by many responsibilities and duties. The more they feel boxed in, the more they may turn to food for a release; they may abandon themselves to eating. This image provides a substitute abandonment—and also sends your spirits soaring—by allowing you to completely let go.

Picture yourself standing out doors on a warm summer afternoon. The sky is bright blue, with large fluffy clouds drifting overhead. What are you wearing? What else do you see in this pleasant outdoor scene? Fill in all of the details, giving color, sound, and sight to your image. Now you notice a trampoline sitting out on the grass. It has an aluminum frame which glints as the sun hits it. Stretched across this frame is a beige-colored canvas cloth. You go over to investigate it. Climb up on the trampoline. Begin to jump up and down on it. Feel the mild sensation of flight, of unrestraint, as you begin to bounce. Experience the liberating, flying sensation as you bounce higher and higher. Allow yourself to enjoy the freedom of the wind rushing past you as you bounce even higher. You are enjoying the feeling and looking about you at the scene below as you bounce higher and higher. You can now bounce high above the trees. You can almost touch the fluffy white clouds above you. Look at the way the trees and houses look as you surge upward.

Spend as much time as you wish, going higher and higher in the air, feeling freer and freer. Enjoy the sensation. Look at the sights. Let go. Just let go and allow your body to experience the motion, the pleasure, and the physical sensations that come with total release and freedom.

Complete the meta-image in any way you like. Go higher, into the clouds, wave at the birds, sing, whatever you wish. Stay as long as you like. Come down off of the trampoline when you are finished. Continue to experience the "high" feeling of the trip.

This image can be a potent release. When you feel boxed in you also feel out of control, which may cause you to indulge in uncontrolled eating. This image provides a letting go, an abandonment in which you are in control.

You might use this trip any time you feel out of control, down, lacking, or depressed. It counteracts the negative feelings. It provides an actual physical feeling of release.

If you truly get into this trip, there is no way you can come back and feel depressed—you have to be exhilarated.

23

CHANGING YOUR THINKING

INTERNAL TAPE RECORDER

Purpose: We all carry old "tapes" in our heads that feed us negative, irrational beliefs. This trip lets you "hear" some of the old tapes, and change them.

※

Picture your head, your hair, your face and neck. When you have the image firmly, move up to your forehead and behind your eyes. It is comfortable, dark and warm in there. Experience how that feels to you. Now image a tape recorder in your head. On it is a reel marked "old tape." Push a button and the old tape plays. The tape begins to play back a situation. You are a child sitting at a dinner table with your family. Relive where you sit, who is there—the total situation. Experience eating dinner in this setting. What is the conversation? What is being said to you? What do you answer? Listen carefully to what you are saying. Complete the scene. When you have finished, push the off button and the tape stops. Remove the old tape. As you do, watch it drop to the floor, unwind, and get tangled up. You realize it is worthless and you throw it in the garbage. Experience your feelings as you do.

Insert a new tape—one that can help you better cope with that eating situation. Rerun the scene with the new tape instead of the old one. Pay attention to the dialogue and conversation in this scene. Allow the scene to continue until the tape has completely wound to the other reel. Then shut off the machine.

For each undesirable tape you hear, try writing a counter tape. Then in real situations when you hear the old tape in your head begin playing, stop the tape recorder immediately and replace the outmoded tape with the new one you've written. You can often become more aware of your own tapes by trying to identify other people's tapes and their resulting behavior.

MAGIC ECHO

Purpose: This trip reveals to you how you really feel or think about yourself, and what you are doing or planning to do at any moment. If you use it when you feel an urge to start bingeing, you may discover that internally you would rather do something other than eat.

❧❧

Picture yourself standing at one end of a long corridor. Call down the corridor, "Hey, you, is that really you?" You hear your question bounce and reverberate down the corridor. Now you hear an answer coming all the way back from the end of the long hall. Listen to the answer. Now call out: "What do you really want right now?" Hear the answer come back like a great echo. Again call out, "Hey, you, do you feel good inside yourself right now?" And wait for the answer. Now ask, "What could you do now to make yourself feel good?" Repeat this last question several times until you get several responses.

❧❧

So many times we eat out of a misplaced desire. We are not really hungry but we want some satisfaction which we cannot pinpoint. We often eat because we literally cannot think of other things we could do to give us as much or more pleasure. Eating has become the habitual response. In our program when we ask people to list pleasurable activities besides eating, most come up with a very short list. But as they lose weight and feel better about themselves, their lists expand.

This trip will help you discover more pleasurable alternatives to eating. Write down the activities you find give you pleasure, and use them also as self-rewards.

FOOD-SPEAK

Purpose: This is a very simple, effective trip in which you carry on a dialogue with food. You may learn

how you feel about what the food is doing to you—
or for you—and why it seems so compelling. It's best
to choose a food that you believe contributes importantly to your weight problem.

❦

Picture a food in front of you that you consider
a problem. Give this food the ability to speak to you.
Ask it, "What do you want from me?" The food answers. What does it say to you? Any answer that
comes to mind is acceptable. Continue to ask more
questions and listen to the answers. Continue the
discussion until you are satisfied that a complete and
honest dialogue has taken place.

❦

After doing this trip, you may want to write
down some of the dialogue and analyze it. It may
offer some startling insights. One man in our program reported that when he did this imagery the first
answer from the food was, "I want to destroy you."
Surprised, he replied, "I don't believe you." The food
then said, "Yes, I want to kill you." He really heard
it for the first time, and realized he had to face the
truth that the food *was* killing him. He considers this
internal dialogue a turning point for him.

SKYWRITING

Purpose: Sometimes you may want to say something
to someone, but can't bring yourself to do it. This
meta-image, in which you write a particular sentence or phrase in the sky for the world to see, acts
as a "rehearsal," making it easier for you to speak up
in real life.

Picture an upcoming situation in which you would like to say something which you find difficult —perhaps something you have wanted to say for a long time. Image the situation until you have the phrase or sentence clearly in mind. Then proceed to a small airfield. It is a warm summer day, with blue sky and no clouds. You are walking toward a hangar where a skywriting plane is kept. As you approach the hangar you see someone wheeling out the plane. Walk up to the plane and notice the bright colors and painted numbers on its side. Feel the hard asphalt under your feet as you stand on the taxiway. Begin to climb into the plane. You feel your muscles stretch as you climb onto the wing and swing yourself into the cockpit. Feel your body sink into the upholstered seat. What does the cockpit feel like, look like, smell like?

When you are ready to take off, pull the starter. As you do, the engine comes to life with a reassuring, sturdy roar. You push in the throttle and the plane gains momentum as you move down the runway. In a few seconds you are airborne, and the scenery is below you. Experience the exhilaration of being lifted in flight. Enjoy the freedom of being up in the blue sky on a lovely cloudless day. Notice the houses, the people, the toylike cars. Soar through the air, feeling free and unencumbered.

Now, activate the mechanism that will release the white smoke with which you will write your message across the sky. Turn this way and that as you form the words in big, bold letters across the sky for all to see. Enjoy the sight as you fly away from the area and see the message clearly outlined in white against the bright-blue sky. Read the message. Notice that people below are reading your message. They seem to approve of it. You fly lower and they smile and wave at you. You smile and wave back and feel wonderful.

Skywrite your message across the sky many times until it seems familiar and comfortable for you. Reflect on the message and the reaction of the observers on the ground to it. Now begin to return to the airfield. You can see where the green grassy field ends and the asphalt strip begins. Effortlessly and joyously, you aim for the airstrip. Feel yourself coming down, closer and closer, descending pleasantly. Feel the slight jolt as the plane wheels hit the runway. You pull back on the throttle and the plane glides to a stop. Experience the enjoyment of a job well done.

❧

Your message could be food-related. For example, some people just have trouble saying "no" when offered food, for fear they will offend. Or it could be anything else you want to say. Sometimes, stifling the impulse to express yourself assertively contributes to a personality picture of yourself that encourages overeating.

Writing the message in the sky, of course, is an antecedent to actually saying it. To get more comfortable, you can also practice saying it aloud, even watching yourself in a mirror say it aloud. The more familiar and natural it begins to sound, the more comfortable you will feel about actually saying it. Many of our clients find that when they do actually get it out, it does not bring nearly the negative reaction they had dreaded. It is probably much more frightening in your mind than in reality.

BODY TALK

Purpose: When you are about to eat something, if you stop to consider whether your "hunger" is legitimate, you may decide it isn't. Thus, if you feel a desire to eat, before doing so or before continuing to eat compulsively, close your eyes and engage in this dialogue imagery.

Picture your stomach with a mouth. It starts to talk and tell you all the reasons you should start eating or continue to eat. Listen to all its arguments attentively. Now picture the upper part of your head or your brain. Give it a mouth. It begins to give its opinion of whether you should eat. Let it speak fully and freely. Listen carefully. Let the head and stomach talk back and forth until you have heard all the reasoning and arguments for each side. After both the stomach and head have had their say, decide what you want to do.

You'll find that given a chance, your head can sometimes talk you out of overeating. And you'll discover by its specious arguments that your stomach really isn't hungry. Its hunger is a phantom. Some people have their stomachs and head engage in lengthy dialogues. But if you get used to imaging such body talk before you eat, you can do it quickly enough to often forestall overeating. Some people when they feel the urge to eat say silently to their stomach with some irritation, "What do you want this time?" Then they instantly consult their head for a counter-opinion.

Of course, lots of times you've probably already said to yourself, "I know I shouldn't eat." But that statement doesn't have the same impact as a structured debate between stomach and head. Sometimes, just while you are conducting a fast discussion, the urge to eat passes.

MESSAGE T-SHIRT

Purpose: This meta-image will help you discover what statements you are making to yourself that could be detrimental to weight loss, and to come up with positive self-statements that will encourage weight loss.

Picture yourself looking in a mirror. You are wearing a T-shirt. On the front of the T-shirt you see a self-slogan, one that you say to yourself often. It is a negative, self-defeating slogan that you often say to yourself about the way you look or feel. Take a moment to fully experience the message on the front of the shirt.

Now turn around. In the mirror you see a slogan on the back of your T-shirt. It is the exact opposite of the statement on the front. It is positive, self-boosting. It makes you feel good. Experience the message on the back of your shirt.

What shows up on the T-shirt is what you are saying to yourself at some level of awareness. To help diminish these negative thoughts, you can image several T-shirts, each with a negative slogan on the front, and a directly opposite positive slogan on the back. Then if you hear yourself parroting one of the negative statements, flip over the T-shirt in your mind and read the positive slogan. Say it repeatedly until it begins to take the place of the negative statement. You will find yourself beginning to act on the positive self-statement instead of the negative, self-defeating one.

24

FEELING GOOD ABOUT YOURSELF

UP SCENE

Purpose: One reason people turn to food is that they feel bad about themselves. This trip is a surefire way of picking yourself up when you feel down. It is a general "up" image in which you develop a detailed mood-raising scene that works for you.

※※

Picture a scene in the past or present in which you really felt good—one in which you really felt high on *you*. It might be a scene based on an emotional high point, a place, an activity, or an accomplishment that made you feel really good.

Now put yourself there. Recreate the experience. What are you doing? Saying? Feeling? Who, if anybody, is there with you? What are they doing? Saying? How are they acting? Be specific about details. Once you have the scene firmly in mind, rerun it entirely. Put yourself into the experience fully. Enjoy it, enjoy feeling up. Do not let anything intrude into your scene about which you have the slightest anxiety or conflict. Make it a scene of pure, total enjoyment.

Since this trip is highly individualistic, there are few instructions for its development. Just be sure to include vivid details, and practice it often, until you know it so well you can recall it in exactly the same way without confusion, especially when you feel your control over your eating slipping. Some people in our program use their "up" scene as a regular part of their daily activity, like brushing their teeth.

The important point is to have it ready in your repertory of "feeling good" meta-images so you can pull it out instantly when you need it.

BRAVO FOR ME

Purpose: Unfortunately, some people are not able to see or accept that they do many things well. Or they feel these things are not very important. But they are. Successful weight control grows on little successes, and begins when you recognize that the smallest steps you take on your behalf can make you feel good, successful, and positive. Acknowledging small successes teaches the "success habit," and contributes to a positive self-image. In this meta-image, you practice recognizing and feeling good about everyday things that you do well. It is adapted from an idea in *Being and Caring* by Victor Daniels and Laurence J. Horowitz.

Picture a television set on which you are going to rerun the day (use the previous day if you do the trip in a morning). Turn the set on and watch your day begin to be rerun on the TV screen. Pay attention to every small activity you were engaged in since you awoke. Pay particular attention to activities that you did well; those you did with ease, with style and flair, and that you enjoyed doing or were comfortable with. It could be something as simple as the way your hands looked as they flew over the typewriter keys or the way you knotted your tie. Or the things can be food-related. For example, the way you held a sandwich, what your hands looked like when you poured your coffee or the way you stirred it, the delicate way you sliced a piece of fruit or the way you look holding a drink. It could be a pleasant conversation you had with somebody. Did you do something nice for someone, or did someone do something nice for you? Did you get or give a smile or a laugh? When did you feel good during the day and why?

Now the show ends. The credits are being shown: Producer, director, actor. Every name is yours. Congratulate yourself on how well you have accomplished these tasks. Say, "Bravo for me!" Appreciate the small successes, and if you can, hear other people applauding or see them patting you on the back. Say to yourself, "I did that well."

❈

Most people find this trip a very positive experience. You may feel a little foolish or peculiar at first, being proud of small accomplishments. But remember that all success comes in minute-by-minute small doses. On the day after doing the trip, watch for the things that you imaged. Recall how well you did them and say that you are going to increase doing little things well until you can say "Bravo for me" very often. In fact, when you do something well, repeat the phrase silently or out loud to yourself as a reward. You'll be surprised how good it makes you feel.

MERRY CHRISTMAS

Purpose: Most people do not give themselves enough "gifts" every day. This trip is designed to encourage self-gift-giving, and help you discover which kinds of things you like, so you can use them to reward yourself.

❈

Picture Christmas Eve. You are alone, and the house is quiet and peaceful. The time is midnight. All of a sudden, Santa Claus is standing in front of you. Picture the Santa Claus, in his outfit. You are a bit startled and amused by his appearing. He begins to talk with you. He says he has brought an enormous bag with him, and there are things in it for you. He produces the bag. It is large and has a faintly leathery smell to it. You ask why he is doing this. He replies that the bag is full of things you might like. Some of these things are material, some are activities, some are half-remembered wishes. He holds out a large package to you, smiling a soft, knowing smile. The package is a white box, wrapped with ribbon and tied with an enormous bow on which is tied a Christmas ornament. You thank him, and begin to open the box. Experience what you find in the box. Take your time. Enjoy it. If it is a material thing, take it out of the box, and use it, put it on, work it, etc. If it isn't material, experience it in some positive way. You find yourself enormously pleased with the "gift" and say so. Santa now hands you another box. Notice how this one is wrapped. Open it, and enjoy what is in it. Open as many boxes as you wish. When you are finished, open your eyes.

❧

Notice what kinds of things showed up in your packages. Were they material? Or were they activities you could participate in? Did they involve other people? Were they small ways of being nice to yourself? Are they gifts you can realistically give to yourself? Make a list of these self-gifts or keep them firmly in mind. Then when you eat in a way you are proud of, reward yourself immediately with one. Do it right then or in a reasonably short time for greatest effectiveness. Though it is important to hold a long-range weight-loss goal in mind—for example, a mind-picture of a thinner you—you also need little rewards as the way to spur you on.

If you find "empty" boxes, as a few have, you probably have been starving yourself psychically and need to try to identify things that please you. You can do that by noticing during the day small things that give you pleasure.

YOUR OWN BEST FRIEND

Purpose: To help you get used to the concept that you should treat yourself as well as you would a valued friend. Some people with weight problems find it easier to feel and act more positively to others than to themselves.

✣

Picture your best friend. Notice the qualities that make this person a best friend. Image a situation when you were with this best friend. Picture the way you treat this person. What do you say? What do you do for the person? How do you speak to him or her? How do you deal with this special friend's needs and wants? How do you settle disagreements that come up with the friend?

Now ask yourself, "Do I treat myself the same way?" Repeat the imaging of how you treat a best friend. Except this time, see yourself as the recipient. Image doing all the things for yourself that you would do for a best friend.

✣

Many people are surprised to find that they do more for others and allow others a wider range of acceptable behavior than they allow themselves. Sometimes putting yourself last develops a habit of self-denial in many areas, often resulting in overeating.

When you treat yourself as a good friend, you

become the one you care about most. That is as it should be. This is not being selfish; it is simply being respectful of yourself. After doing this trip, resolve to treat yourself more positively, with respect, care, understanding, and acceptance. Also try the trip using different friends to get a wider range of responses. If you notice that you are denigrating yourself, flash a "best friend" image in your mind. Think of it constantly, and it will do wonders for your self-respect.

TESTIMONIAL DINNER

Purpose: It's often not easy for people to think of good things about themselves, and harder yet to accept and acknowledge compliments. In this trip, you acknowledge that there are many worthwhile things to be said for you that you should feel good about.

Picture yourself at a testimonial dinner, and *you* are the guest of honor. People have come here to speak about your good qualities. Experience the scene. Who is there? What are you wearing? What are you feeling?

A speaker is introduced. He or she begins a speech, saying some wonderful things about you, what a worthwhile person you are. What the person says makes you feel good because you know the speaker's feelings are genuine. Listen to the speech all the way through.

A second speaker is introduced who also says some very nice things he or she feels about you. Other speakers rise to pay tributes to you. Listen to everyone and don't contradict them. Recognize that the things they say are true. Now, you stand and all of the people smile and applaud. Enjoy the scene for a little while, then allow it to slowly fade out.

❧

After the trip, it will be interesting to think about who spoke for you. Were you comfortable with what they were saying? Usually the comments reflect the traits that you personally regard as most important. Interestingly, our clients report that the one thing they usually don't notice at their testimonial dinner is the food. As one said, "I wasn't the least bit interested in it; something better was going on for me." That's true; when you feel good about yourself food becomes less important as a way of consoling yourself.

This is a scene you can play back whenever you are feeling low, or perhaps when tempted to try to improve your mood by eating.

CENTERING

Purpose: To help you get to the core of yourself, and to feel at peace. This is a trip that will give you a great feeling of calm. You can use it for feeling good in general or as a help in reducing eating, especially when you are alone.

❧

Hear your name being called. It sounds pleasant and friendly. Say your name to yourself over and over, again and again. As you hear your name a pleasant image comes to mind, some thought or memory. Allow yourself to fully experience this pleasant memory or thought.

Now you are at the head of a staircase. The staircase has five steps that will take you to the center of who you are, to your core of self. At the center are the answers. There you can work out your eating problems. Count the steps as you move deeper and deeper into yourself. Five, beginning . . . four, getting closer . . . three, deeper and deeper . . . two, still closer and more deeply centered . . . one, centered and at peace. Say your name to yourself here and allow the good feeling to flow into you. Tell yourself that you have the ability to work out your eating problems, and you will. As you center, you know the answers are inside of you. You know what is best for you. Think about the answers.

25

FINDING MORE ANSWERS

YOU'RE THE DOCTOR

Purpose: This trip dramatically demonstrates that you can evaluate your own progress and, based on that, prescribe for yourself what more you need to do. It helps you create a specific list of things to do to aid you in long-range weight control. This trip is meant to organize your plans for the future after you have read and tried a number of other meta-images in the book.

🌿

Picture yourself in a physician's office. You are there to obtain a prescription that will result in proper eating and weight loss. Notice that there is a large desk in the room, many books and journals, chairs, diplomas of many sorts. Image all of the details. What color are the walls painted? What kind of furniture is in the room? Is it a small and cozy consultation room, or large and imposing? What do the drapes and carpeting look like? What is on the desk?

When you have fully created the scene, place yourself behind the desk, where the physician sits. Feel yourself lower your body into the comfortable chair. Fold your hands across the top of the desk, lean slightly forward, and call for the nurse to bring in the next patient. The door opens, and you walk in. Ask yourself to sit down. Note that you have made much progress and that, together, you will work out some important solutions to your weight problem. Note that, together, you will develop a prescription for the future.

Experience you, the patient, in a dialogue with you, the physician. As the physician, you ask the kind of questions that help pinpoint constructive behavior and attitudes. You note that progress has indeed been made. As the patient, you help answer questions, and actively engage in developing a prescription for yourself for the future. Allow yourself to experience whatever dialogue develops. As you both talk, you evolve a specific prescription for future behavior that will help you to be of normal weight. The doctor writes each thing down on a pad. Continue until you are satisfied with the future prescription. Then take the paper, thank the doctor, and leave the office.

※

Many of our clients say this meta-image definitely helps them clarify the steps they yet need to take to permanent weight control. It can also help identify blocks or "hidden" impediments to progress.

For example, the dialogue between you the physician and you the patient may illuminate internal conflicts or resistance.

We suggest that after the imagery, you write the prescription out clearly, and analyze each element of it carefully. Note beside each recommendation what you think the benefit of carrying it out would be. That way, you can define the payoff, and determine whether you think it is worth acting on.

QUESTIONS AND ANSWERS

Purpose: To give you a technique by which you can get future answers to your weight-loss problems.

Picture yourself in a classroom. Make it one in which you have been successful and enjoyed yourself. In this room, we, the authors, will be your teachers. Picture either or both of us in your classroom. Picture what we look like, where we are sitting or standing, what our voices sound like. Now describe to us some weight-control problem you are working on. Ask us questions about what to do. Hear us answer you. Then resolve to act on the answers. Picture us smiling and praising you. See us congratulating you.

The theory of this trip is that if you have read this book and done a number of the meta-images, your mind has stored up a great deal of knowledge about how to solve your own weight problem. You have the creative solutions inside you. By asking us you merely release your own creative solutions.

One of Dr. Stern's college students uses this technique in a slightly different way. While taking a test the student goes into her head, and images asking Dr. Stern the answers. Dr. Stern tells her and she writes them down. The student used to get C's. Since she started using this technique, she gets A's.

26

CONSTRUCT YOUR OWN MIND TRIPS

After you do a number of the mind trips, you might want to make up some of your own to fit your individual situation. In fact, you may find that you can't help creating new trips or improvising on those in the book; often they just begin to present themselves to your mind automatically as ways of dealing with problems of all types. Many people in our program have come up with ingenious and bizarre trips they find helpful.

One man who was virtually living off tranquilizers decided to see what would happen if he instead imaged taking the tranquilizers. He closed his eyes, went through all the motions of swallowing the pills, and waited. He experienced the same kind of calm as when he actually took tranquilizers—and now takes them entirely in his mind.

A woman who lost 40 pounds routinely using the mind trips improvised on Jungle Doors. When she is annoyed with someone, she puts them behind the door and slams it in their face. She takes great delight in imaging the door striking her boss's nose as it slams shut. By putting what is bothering her behind the doors, she is able to put her feelings temporarily out of the way also. Previously, she used to express her frustration by drinking Scotch.

Another woman, when she is tempted to eat, images her own funeral. She sees herself lying in the coffin. The most embarrassing part of the scene for her is when the pallbearers try to pick up her casket and carry it from the church. They stagger under the weight.

Examine your own situation to see what new meta-images might work for you. Sharpen your observations of what you and others say. Often figures of speech give clues to how you are feeling, which you can develop into mind trips. One woman with three small children used to binge in the late afternoons. She finally heard herself say, "I'm stuck in the house." She developed an image of actually being "stuck" to a large piece of fly paper, from which she managed eventually to escape.

Let your imagination run free; unleash the power of your own mind, your own images. You can do or be whatever you want. You've learned how; now you can make it happen.

Related Readings

Assagioli, Roberto. *Psycho-Synthesis: A Manual of Principles and Techniques.* New York: Hobbs, Droman, 1965.

Bruno, Frank, J. *Think Yourself Thin.* New York: Barnes & Noble, 1973.

Carper, Jean, and Krause, Patricia A. *All in One Calorie Counter.* New York: Bantam Books, 1974.

Ellis, Albert, and Harper, Robert A. *A Guide to Rational Living.* Englewood Cliffs, N. J.: Prentice-Hall, 1961.

Ferguson, James M. *Learning to Eat: Behavior Modification for Weight Control.* Palo Alto, Calif.: Bull Publishing Co., 1975.

Hendricks, Gay, and Wills, Russel. *The Centering Book: Awareness Activities for Children, Parents and Teachers.* Englewood Cliffs, N. J.: Prentice Hall, 1975.

Lazarus, Arnold, and Fay, Allan. *I Can If I Want To.* New York: William Morrow & Co., 1975.

Mahoney, Michael J., and Mahoney, Kathryn. *Permanent Weight Control—A Total Solution to the Dieter's Dilemma.* New York: Norton, 1976.

————, and Thoreson, Carl E. *Self Control: Power to the Person.* Belmont, Calif.: Brooks/Cole, 1974.

Maltz, Maxwell. *Psycho-Cybernetics.* New York: Pocket Books, 1969.

Masters, Robert, and Houston, Jean. *Mind Games.* New York: Viking, 1972.

Sheehan, Peter. *The Function and Nature of Imagery.* New York: Academic Press, 1972.

Shorr, Joseph E. *Psycho-Imagination Therapy.* New York: Intercontinental Medical Books, 1972.

Singer, Jerome L. *Imagery and Daydream Methods in Psychotherapy and Behavior Modification.* New York: Academic Press, 1974.

————. *The Inner World of Daydreaming.* New York: Harper & Row, 1975.

Smith, Adam. *Powers of Mind.* New York: Random House, 1975.

Stuart, Richard B, and Davis, Barbara. *Slim Chance in a Fat World.* Champaign, Ill.: Research Press, 1972.

Watson, David L., and Tharp, Roland G. *Self-Directed Behavior: Self Modification for Personal Adjustment.* Belmont, Calif.: Brooks/Cole, 1972.

Wolpe, Joseph. *The Practice of Behavior Therapy.* Long Island City, N. Y.: Pergamon Press, 1969.

————, and Lazarus, Arnold. *Behavior Therapy Techniques.* Long Island City, N. Y.: Pergamon Press, 1966.

The Best in Historical Romance from Playboy Paperbacks

DIANA SUMMERS
- ___16502 **LOVE'S WICKED WAYS** $2.25
- ___16450 **WILD IS THE HEART** $1.95

RACHEL COSGROVE PAYES
- ___16592 **BRIDE OF FURY** $2.50
- ___16546 **THE COACH TO HELL** $2.25
- ___16481 **MOMENT OF DESIRE** $1.95

NORAH HESS
- ___16459 **CALEB'S BRIDE** $1.95
- ___16371 **ELISHA'S WOMAN** $1.95
- ___16454 **HUNTER'S MOON** $1.95
- ___16671 **MARNA** $2.50

BARBARA BONHAM
- ___16470 **DANCE OF DESIRE** $1.95
- ___16638 **THE DARK SIDE OF PASSION** $2.50
- ___16399 **PASSION'S PRICE** $1.95
- ___16345 **PROUD PASSION** $1.95

A MARVELOUS SELECTION
OF TOP-NOTCH MYSTERY THRILLERS
FOR YOUR READING PLEASURE

PHILLIPS LORE

___16587	**WHO KILLED THE PIE MAN?**	$1.75
___16694	**THE LOOKING GLASS MURDERS**	$1.95
___16652	**MURDER BEHIND CLOSED DOORS**	$1.95

MICHAEL COLLINS

___16551	**BLUE DEATH**	$1.75
___16506	**SHADOW OF A TIGER**	$1.50
___16525	**THE SILENT SCREAM**	$1.50
___16478	**WALK A BLACK WIND**	$1.50
___16593	**ACT OF FEAR**	$1.75
___16672	**THE BRASS RAINBOW**	$1.95

MARGOT ARNOLD

___16639	**CAPE COD CAPER**	$1.95
___16534	**EXIT ACTORS, DYING**	$1.75
___16684	**ZADOK'S TREASURE**	$1.95

CHARLES ALVERSON

| ___16530 | **GOODEY'S LAST STAND** | $1.95 |
| ___16603 | **NOT SLEEPING, JUST DEAD** | $1.95 |

MICHAEL P. HODEL &
SEAN M. WRIGHT

| ___16711 | **ENTER THE LION** | $2.50 |

PLAYBOY PAPERBACKS
Book Mailing Service
P.O. Box 690 Rockville Centre, New York 11571

NAME _____

ADDRESS _____

CITY _____ STATE _____ ZIP _____

Please enclose 50¢ for postage and handling if one book is ordered;
25¢ for each additional book. $1.50 maximum postage and handling
charge. No cash, CODs or stamps. Send check or money order.

Total amount enclosed: $ _____

From Playboy Paperbacks, novels guaranteed to entertain, delight and captivate you

PLAYBOY NOVELS OF HORROR AND THE OCCULT
ABSOLUTELY CHILLING